The <u>WRITE</u> Way
to <u>BETTER</u> E.M.S.

How to Organize, Write
& Give Better E.M.S. Reports

By Walter C. Kennedy, Jr., M.Ed., EMT-P

toExcel

San Jose New York Lincoln Shanghai

The Write Way to Better E.M.S.

How To Organize, Write and Give Better E.M.S. Reports

Published by toExcel
an imprint of iUniverse.com, Inc.

For information address:
iUniverse.com, Inc.
620 North 48th Street
Suite 201
Lincoln, NE 68504-3467
www.iuniverse.com

ISBN: 0-595-00424-5

Printed in the United States of America

To my Mom & Dad, two fine people
who have always had faith in me.

Table of Contents

Acknowledgements vii
Disclaimer ix
Introduction 1

Section 1: Developing a Clear, Concise Report

1   *Scenes from EMS* 5
2   *Goals* 9
3   *Purpose, Form, and Content of Written Reports* 11
4   *Reporting Format* 15
5   *The Simplified EMS (SEMS) Format* 19
6   *The Report as a Resource in the Hospital* 41
7   *Ambulance-to-Hospital Radio Communication* 45
8   *Presenting the Case in the Emergency Department* 51
9   *Special Reporting Situations* 55
10 *Final Remarks* 79

Section 2: Sample Run Reports & Classroom Exercises

11 *Run Report Forms* 83
12 *Classroom Exercises* 159
A   *Common Deficiencies in Report Writing* 177
B   *105 CMR 170.240 Records* 179
C   *Process for Investigating Complaints* 181
D   *Terms* 183
E   *Commonly-Used Abbreviations* 185
F   *Charting Symbols* 195
    End Notes 197
    Index 205

Acknowledgements

This book is the product of many people, and a number of thanks are in order. Marianne, Sean, Kyle, and Brendan have had to tolerate the long hours I spent at the keyboard. The process of taking the material and placing it in usable form was greatly assisted by Doug Wilcox at WordSmith, whose many hours spent in setup and design helped make this textbook possible. The insights provided by Tom Kennedy and the technology available at Cor-Print have helped with the physical production of the book.

I appreciate the opportunity to have interviewed Anna Sinclair, M.D., attending physician at Quincy Hospital, who provided a physician's perspective of prehospital EMS reports in the emergency department; Paul Coffey, Director of Basic EMT Training, and Michael Pichon, both of the Massachusetts Office of Emergency Medical Services, who provided information about the reporting process throughout Massachusetts; and Robert Tinker of the Boston Police Department Training Academy for his invaluable assistance and expert counsel on the topic of crime scene management.

The information gathering for the classroom exercises accomplished by Ruth Stokes saved me much time and effort.

Proofreading is a time-consuming process. I received many useful comments and suggestions for improvement from a number of people who gave their time to help me with this textbook.

For this help, I would like to thank Peter Moyer, M.D., Director of the Emergency Department at Boston City Hospital and Chair of Emergency Medicine at Boston University School of Medicine; Ralph Warren, M.D., Attending Physician in the Emergency Department, Assistant in Surgery, and Assistant in Medicine, Massachusetts General Hospital, and Instructor in Surgery at Harvard Medical School; Alan Hildreth King, Attorney at Law, Member of the Massachusetts Department of Public Health, Office of Emergency Medical Services Executive Board, and Chairman of the Peer Review Committee; Ed Pike, Attorney at Law, EMT, and Jami L. Freeman, EMT, who, in addition to proofreading, have field tested the principles presented in the text.

A special thanks to Diane Shannon Gray, BA, Public Relations Specialist, D.S.G. Designs, for laboriously ensuring proper grammar and usage throughout the text.

Disclaimer

This book is sold with the understanding that the author and the publisher are not engaged in giving legal, accounting, or other professional service. If legal or other expert assistance or advice is required, the services of a competent professional should be sought.

This book is intended to be used as a guide. Local protocols and standards should be followed. Any discrepancies should be referred to your medical or administrative director for clarification.

This text uses cases as a learning tool. It bases the cases themselves and the medical conditions described on situations that have occurred in the prehospital setting. However, facts presented in these cases have been significantly altered in order to protect the privacy of the individuals involved.

This text uses an example of a report form that contains information the author considers necessary to an effective report form. The specific form any individual EMS system uses may vary in style. The author recommends that readers be familiar with the form their own system uses. The form that the text presents is a guide.

Introduction

This textbook presents a method of organizing, writing, and giving reports in emergency medical service. It recounts the various reporting formats that health care professionals use. It then describes a format versatile enough for use when organizing and presenting the case via radio, in person, or in writing. It also is useful to keep the patient interview and history-taking organized in what I call the Simplified Emergency Medical Services (SEMS) format. The text offers guidance on presenting the patient to triage and other emergency department staff, and on writing a patient care report. It also lends guidance on how to give radio notifications.

The text identifies and presents discussion of situations that commonly present to EMTs and paramedics. The book discusses issues surrounding consent, refusals, Do Not Resuscitate Orders (DNRs) and sudden death. The section on crime scene management will help both the EMT/paramedic and the police officer. Also included are sections concerning child and elder abuse.

The Classroom Exercises section uses cases to strengthen the reporting skills of the EMT and the paramedic. The exercises provide the chance to practice giving reports using the skills presented in the text.

The textbook is written for the present, when pen and paper are the essential tools for the EMS report. The future holds promise for the use of high technology information systems. Such systems could include computer consoles in the ambulance. These consoles might accept typed or written reports directly from the field. It is possible the day will come when voice-activated systems allow dictation of the report by the EMT or paramedic directly into the information system with hard copy retrievable on an as-needed basis. Whatever changes take place, a format will still be needed. The SEMS format will keep you organized whether writing on a clipboard or dictating into a machine.

The book is a foundation. Build on it. Mastery of skills requires the provider to practice the principles with every report that he gives or writes. Only then will good reporting skills become a habit.

Section 1

Developing a Clear, Concise Report

1

Scenes from EMS

Scene One

It is 2200 hours (10:00 p.m.). One more hour and the shift will be over. The evening has been rather busy with a cardiac arrest, a heroin overdose, and a shooting. Then there were two "man down" calls that turned out to be police matters, and three other calls you were cancelled on before you arrived at the scene.

Just as you make another attempt to eat a cold supper, the dispatcher assigns you to a motor vehicle accident reported with injuries. So much for the meal.

The response takes only a couple of minutes. You arrive to find the police on scene with a driver who they think is intoxicated. As you approach, you hear the driver say to the officer, "...what d'ya think I am? Dunk er sumptum?" He apparently failed to negotiate a turn and now has a street lamp as a hood ornament.

The man is a bit hostile toward you, and does not want you to touch him. He states he does not want to go to a hospital and does not need you. You succeed in getting him to let you take his blood pressure and pulse. You do not see any obvious injuries. Your partner examines the motor vehicle. Although there is rather extensive front end damage, the dashboard and steering wheel appear intact. The windshield is broken but this seems to be more a result of the impact with the street light than any impact from the driver's head.

After a few more attempts to get the man to consent to treatment and transport, which he firmly and loudly refuses, he is left in the custody of the police department.

You clear the scene and return to your quarters to await the end of shift.

Two years later, you're standing in court defending your actions at the accident scene. The man had internal injuries and after a night at the police station he was brought to the emergency department and rushed to surgery. He died in the operating room. His family is suing you, your employer, and the police department.

Your only recollection of the incident is what you wrote down on the run report form and as you take the witness stand, that is what you hold in your hand. Your job and income are on the line as you face the charges of contributing to the man's wrongful death and denying him due process. His estate's attorney claims you were negligent. The run report holds the key to your actions and frame of mind on that night.

Scene Two

It is early Sunday morning on a quiet fall day. The air is crisp, the temperature is comfortable. It has been a busy week. You hope today will be slow. You actually get to read part of the newspaper and to eat breakfast without having to gulp it all down.

The morning solitude is broken by the bell that signals a medical response. Your dispatcher sends you a report of a man down and possibly unconscious in a home on the other side of town. Your response takes about ten minutes.

At the home, you are met by a woman who says her husband is not breathing. She thinks he is dead. You go upstairs to the bedroom and find the man in cardiac arrest, seated in a chair. The woman, his wife, says he was talking to their daughter on the telephone when he became unconscious. She found him like this a few minutes later. The daughter, apparently sensing something was wrong, hung up the phone and called you.

The wife has called the daughter back, spoken with her and informed you that the daughter is now on the way to the house. It has probably been more than twenty minutes since all of this occurred.

After assessing the situation, you determine not to resuscitate the man based on an extended down time. You explain to the wife that nothing can be done, since too much time has elapsed. You collect some information, retrieve your equipment, and leave the scene in the hands of the police. Six months later you are sitting in an administrative hearing at your state's EMS agency. They are seeking to revoke your certification. When they received the complaint from the family, your run report was the first place they looked. They hand you a copy of your report.

Scene Three

You respond to a stabbing incident. The victim is 15 years old, in cardiac arrest, with police officers performing CPR. A rapid assessment reveals a single wound to the abdomen just below the xiphoid. You manage the airway as the patient is rapidly packaged and moved downstairs through a crowd to your ambulance.

It takes a couple of minutes to drive the patient to the trauma center. Based on your history of the incident, a decision is made to discontinue the effort to resuscitate.

Over the next year you are interviewed by homicide detectives, private investigators and have been subpoenaed. Today, you find yourself in court testifying as to your actions at the scene. Another child is charged with murder. There is some question about the weapons evidence on the scene. Your recollection of events is considered important. You are handed your run report as the document you are to refer to concerning the case.

As you can see from the above situations, almost any EMS call can result in a referral to the documentation you created at the time of the incident. These are not the only situations where good documentation becomes important. Long after you have left the patient at the hospital, your written record remains as a source of information about events that occurred in the prehospital setting. As in all other areas of healthcare, thorough documentation is a necessary skill.

The following pages are designed to help you develop those skills.

2
Goals

Why learn about documentation? How necessary is it? If you think about it, most EMS responses require some form of report. The report may be lengthy or short, but some record must exist.

When you are in a program designed to help you develop better skills of any sort, you need to know what the goals are. You can tell if you are making progress by referring to the goals and comparing them to what you have learned.

Not all learning takes place in the classroom. In programs such as this, the learning should also take place in the work environment. EMTs and paramedics should constantly review their reporting techniques. They should keep the good parts and try to make them better, while identifying the poor parts and finding ways to improve them.

The following list of program goals will help you keep track of your learning progress.

- Participants will be able to produce a report written in a clear and concise manner consistent with the principles presented during the program.

- With practice, participants will write clearer and more detailed reports as a result of concepts conveyed during the program.

- Participants will be able to list common deficiencies found in documentation of EMS responses.

- Participants will be able to state the primary purpose of a medical record.

- Participants will be able to recite and define the terms and concepts about types of consent.

- Participants will be able to define and give examples of abandonment.

- Participants will be able to define and give examples of negligence.

- Participants will be able to list four ingredients of a malpractice action as stated in the American Heart Association *Textbook of Advanced Cardiac Life Support.*

- Participants will be able to define and give examples of malpractice.

- Participants will be able to give an oral report to triage in a simulated radio notification environment in a clear and concise manner, consistent with the principles presented during the program.

- Participants will be able to give an oral report to a triage person in a simulated emergency room triage situation in a clear and concise manner, consistent with the principles presented during the program.

- Participants will be able to give an oral report to emergency department personnel in a simulated emergency department situation in a clear and concise manner consistent with the principles presented during the program.

- With practice, participants will present patients to hospital emergency department triage personnel in a clearer, more concise, and organized manner, as a result of concepts conveyed during the program.

- With practice, participants will present patients to hospital emergency department personnel in a clearer and more organized manner and with greater detail, as a result of concepts conveyed during the program.

3

Purpose, Form, and Content of Written Reports

If you didn't write it, you didn't do it.

There are many vital pieces of information included on the written report form.

Written reports provide a permanent record of what occurred during the medical call. Report forms used in prehospital emergency care should provide space for recording the following information:

Space for recording the day of the week and date; the record of the dispatch, arrival, scene departure, hospital arrival and clear times; a mileage record from scene to hospital; the dispatch location, as well as space for noting any changes in the dispatch information. Include a space for the nature code of the call; a space for recording the patient's name, address and telephone number; and the patient's date of birth, age and sex. Include a space for recording the next of kin with address and telephone number.

Include a space for recording vital signs and for writing a narrative. The narrative should include the history and physical findings. A record of advanced life support procedures performed and the time of the intervention needs inclusion. Also include a record of changes during transport.

A record of the response unit identification number must appear. Identify the physician giving medical control. The form also needs space for the signatures of the EMTs or paramedics.[1,2]

Many systems employ check-off boxes for some of the patient assessment and treatment

Remember that you are writing a legal document.

You are usually the only person who sees the patient when the illness or injuy happened. You need to tell the hospital staff about what you saw.

information. Some use check-off boxes to show non-transport situations and to record the presence of other agencies on the call.

The form itself has use as a medical record, for research and statistical purposes, and as a legal document. It also may contain space for billing information. A copy should be available to become part of the patient's medical record at the hospital.

The EMT/paramedic sees the patient in the environment where the illness or injury occurs. He is usually the only member of the health care team with this perspective. Thus, EMTs and paramedics are in a unique position. Valuable information concerning mechanisms of injury, patient lifestyle and living environment is available to the trained observer. Written reports provide a means of passing on the information gained from this unique perspective. It makes it available to the other health care professionals who will give care to the patient.

For instance, many ill or injured persons require admission to an intensive care unit. Questions will arise concerning what happened to the patient. The unit personnel will spend time trying to trace the steps of the patient back through the system. They will need to find out information that is already available on the well-written EMS report form.[3] The form provides a mechanism for continuity of patient care.[4,5] Your report must relate your findings and treatment in a clear, legible way.

EMS personnel need to make sure that other medical professionals, such as those who work in hospitals, know about the existance of prehospital care reports. The reports are a resource for them, but only if they know about them, receive them, and read them. This means the EMS report must become part of the patient's medical record.

From a medical-legal standpoint, the report provides a record of the physical findings and the care given. It also may contain information about circumstances surrounding injuries and illnesses. Occasionally, the courts subpoena EMTs and paramedics. The court asks them to provide testimony about their actions and observations at a case. This can occur even though their conduct is not specifically in question. In cases such as these a poorly documented response would leave the credibility of the EMT or paramedic open to question.[6]

Liability and Malpractice

EMTs and paramedics extend the physician to persons having a medical emergency outside the hospital. They hold themselves out to the public as reasonably and responsibly competent providers of care. As such, the public expects them to act responsibly. If the patient or the patient's family perceives the care to be less than reasonableand responsible, they may claim malpractice or negligence has occurred.

The patient has a contract with the emergency medical service. The contractual agreement to provide care begins when the emergency medical service receives the call. This is an implied contract. The patient expects the provider to uphold the contract. The provider does this by giving reasonable care. The provider protects himself by documenting the provision of reasonable care.

The patient (or the representative of the patient) must show four elements to successfully claim malpractice or negligence.

1. The provider had a duty to act.

2. The provider breached the duty.

3. The patient suffered harm.

4. The harm occurred because of the breach of duty.[7]

To show that the patient received adequate care, a review of the provider's actions would take place. The provider needs to act reasonably. What is reasonable? In most cases, expert testimony determines what is reasonable by focusing on care expectations from a reputable provider of similar service in the community.[8]

For example, an emergency medical technician needs to act as another reasonable EMT would act.[9] The same is true for the paramedic. The standard the community holds the EMT/paramedic to is different from that to which it holds the physician. This is because the level of training and experience is different.

To state it another way, you hold yourself out as a provider of emergency care. The state certifies (or licenses) you. It also licenses your employer. The public assumes that you meet minimum standards about training, equipment and the care you give. You have the responsibility to respond to emergency calls. During the response, and when you arrive, you must act responsibly. You must give reasonable care. The care is reasonable if it meets local, regional and national standards for EMS providers at the time the act occured.

The patient must not suffer harm from your care. If the patient suffers harm due to your care, you could be negligent. The patient can charge you with malpractice.

Toward Quality EMS

The trip sheet provides some insight into the quality of the service the EMS system provides. It is certainly not the only measure of quality assurance. It is also subject to manipulation. It does, however, provide insight into the actions and thought processes of field EMTs and paramedics.

It is one of the tools available for building a strong EMS system.

4

Reporting Format

"The primary purpose of the (office) medical record is to document appropriate patient care.[10]"

Consistent with this purpose, the report enhances communication among those who are caring for the patient.[11] Therefore, write the report in a manner understandable by others in the health care field. To help in meeting this criteria, you must use an organized format that allows for a clear and logical flow of information. There are several possible systems or formats that can accomplish this.

Problem Oriented Medical Record

The provider arranges the problem oriented medical record according to each of the patient's problems.[12] It starts with a database that is drawn from a complete history and the physical exam. The person writing the report supplements this with diagnostic tests. After the provider completes this process, a problem list is drawn up. The provider then deals with each problem as an individual entity. Obviously, a system such as this suits the clinic or office setting much better than the prehospital emergency setting. It is lengthy and therefore time consuming, and requires testing that may not be available outside the hospital. The major drawback is the length, which translates into time. In the emergency situation, time is usually the scarce commodity. Development of the detailed information required in the problem-oriented format requires more time than would usually be available.

Source Oriented Record

The provider arranges the source-oriented record according to the source of the information.[13] This method relies on getting information from x-rays, lab reports and progress notes. It is not very useful in the prehospital setting where all such information and sources are usually absent.

S.O.A.P.

Four sections make up this structure:

- *Subjective* findings (chief complaint and present history)

- *Objective* findings (such as physical findings)

- *Assessment*, the documented resolution of the findings

- *Plan* for further diagnostic or therapeutic action.[14]

Use of the "SOAP" structure may have some utility if the patient has only one problem. However, if the patient has more than one problem, then a situation similar to the problem oriented method exists. Each problem requires an individual SOAP note.[15] This report method is better suited to situations in the hospital or clinic. It is particularly useful for nursing notes. It was not designed for the prehospital setting or conditions.

Problem/Source Record

The design of the modified problem/source record combines the best of these two methods. It uses only one set of SOAP headings.[16] Again, this method is lengthy. Because of this, its utility is in the hospital rather than the prehospital setting.

Traditional Write-Up

The traditional write-up makes use of headings followed by a narrative style.[17] This is used by some physicians in the hospital ward. However, it becomes a rather lengthy way of transferring information in the emergency department. It is time consuming to read. Its lengthiness may dissuade physician and nursing staff from reading it, particularly if they need information in a hurry. Since this is exactly the case in the emergency situation, the provider needs a format that is brief but complete.

The physician will already have a familiarity with the traditional write-up. What is needed is to change (or simplify) the write-up to meet the needs of the emergency setting. For example, detailed documenting of family and social history and an in-depth review of systems are unneccesary in most cases. Also, the documenting of impressions and the treatment plan will probably be a bit out of place in the fast pace of prehospital health care. The impression will have already been arrived at, and treatment planned and given, including transport to a hospital, before the case is documented. The other portions of the traditional write-up do have a place in EMS documentation.

5

The Simplified EMS
(SEMS) Format

Think about this for a moment. You, the EMT or paramedic, need the ability to communicate to a variety of people in a clear and concise manner.

First, there is the patient. You need interviewing skills that enable you to focus the conversation on the immediate problem. These skills must elicit the information you need so you can develop a plan for rapid intervention.

You also have to communicate with hospital personnel by radio. This could take the form of a hospital notification. It also could take the form of a detailed conversation with the medical control physician.

When you arrive at the hospital, you must communicate explicity with triage. That means you must avoid conveying information that this individual does not need.

You also need to communicate effectively with the physicians, nurses, and other staff members who will be responsible for actual care of the patient. They need an organized, detailed oral report—and they need it given in a manner which is as clear and concise as possible.

Then, after you do all of this verbally, you need to write a report. That report must be useful in the present situation in the emergency department, and the future situations that could arise in the hospital units and wards.

What you need is a format that will help you organize the patient interview, the hospital notification, and the conversation with medical control. It also has to get you through triage, and help you present the patient condition clearly to the emergency department staff. Then you have to use it to help you organize the written report. You need one format that does it all!

Some texts allude to this type of format.[18,19,20] Rapid information retrieval is the advantage of a simplified (SEMS) format. The SEMS format incorporates some of the headings found in other types of record systems. The hospital staff simply scans the headings to find and retrieve the information. The headings are drawn from the traditional write-up and the problem oriented method. Therefore, they are instantly recognizable by the physician and nursing staff in the hospital. Now you must ensure that the hospital staff finds the correct information under the particular heading.

There is an added benefit to the SEMS format approach. When ambulance-to-hospital radio communication is necessary, you can use the SEMS format. The SEMS format will help keep the ambulance-to-hospital communication organized. This helps the EMT/paramedic in formulating and delivering a clear and concise report. With practice prehospital personnel will present the patient in an organized and efficient manner.

The hospital personnel should be given a clear verbal portrait of the situation. This means avoiding repetition of points and periods of either silence or *ahhh's** as the field person desperately tries to organize his thoughts while pressing the radio transmit switch.

---

* Ahhh's — *sounds made to fill space in conversation not taken up by actual words or phrases.*

Use of the Simplified Format

The headings to be employed when using the SEMS format are:

- Chief Complaint (CC)
- History of Present Illness/Injury (HPI)
- Past Medical History (PMH)
- Physical Examination (PE)
- Treatment Given (Rx)
- Changes During Transport.[21,22,23]

What must be done next is to decide under which heading a particular piece of information belongs. To begin the report, identify the patient characteristics. This is simply the age and sex of the patient. If appropriate to the case, state the patient's racial or ethnic background here, also.

Chief Complaint

This is why the patient called.

The *Chief Complaint* (CC) should include the complaint and the duration of the complaint.[24] This is what the patient states is wrong with them. This is why patients summon the ambulances. This is for what they are seeking treatment. Record it in the patient's own words, with quotation marks, or restructure it to make it clearer. If you restructure it, keep the basic meaning intact. Also note who provided the information. Was it the patient himself, or a relative or friend? It is also helpful to identify and note the language spoken by the patient or the historian.

The chief complaint is primarily a subjective piece of information. Obviously if the patient seeks treatment for a visible laceration, this is the complaint. However, most patients requesting help from EMS have medical rather than surgical complaints. Regardless of whether it is medical or surgical, the chief complaint is still *the reason the patient seeks medical attention.*

Some patients have a major underlying illness. Include it with the chief complaint if such inclusion will lead to immediate understanding of the problem.[25] For instance, consider the patient with altered mental status who is a diabetic. Include this at the outset of the medical report. For the paramedic seeking orders to treat the suspected hypoglycemia, this will help the physician to better understand the field problem. Remember, the physician is directing the paramedic from a remote location. The paramedic must paint a clear picture of the problem for the doctor.

It is possible that the patient's perception of their problem is erroneous. For example, the patient claiming chest pain may indeed have pain (a subjective concept). Further questioning shows that the pain is in fact in the upper abdomen. Still recorded this as chest pain under the chief complaint. This is what the patient presents as the problem. State the true location of the pain under a later heading. The point here is to relate the patient's perception of the problem.

History of Present Illness

This is what has been happening recently. It has to do with how the chief complaint developed.

The *History of Present Illness* (HPI) is the most challenging part of the clinical exam.[26] Here the EMT or paramedic writes out the story behind the chief complaint. This is the part of the medical record that requires a constant refinement of skills. The tendency among EMTs and paramedics is to write either too much or not enough. You also may see this phenomenon among other health care professionals, particularly those used to writing problem-oriented reports in the wards. EMS reports need to be brief and concise. The clinical goal of EMS is to provide emergency care. The documentation should reflect good problem identification and appropriate assessment and intervention.

Some instructors involved in EMS teach EMTs and paramedics not to write very much, or nothing at all. They do this under a mistaken belief. They teach you to write nothing. That way no one can accuse or convict you of wrongdoing or negligence. This is because they believe nothing will exist to support allegations of wrongdoing or negligence.

As is shown elsewhere in this text, nothing could be further from the truth. In fact, this is a dangerous misconception. In the courtroom, if it was not written down on the report form, it was not done.

What to Include, What to Leave Out. Some report writers may include superfluous information. They have the belief you should record *everything*. If the information has relevance, it belongs in the report. If it is irrelevant, it serves only to distract the reader from the task of assimilating the information and drawing a conclusion.

Excessive verbiage is a fault. Happily, practice changes this. This change requires diligence. Omit statements such as "the patient states...". The report is about the patient. Assume that the statements are the patient's unless otherwise noted. A review of many patient reports by EMTs and paramedics shows the use of "patient states..." rapidly becomes excessive, when each statement by the patient is prefaced with "the patient states...". Once should suffice. Organize all the patient statements together, in a logical flow. The report will gain clarity.

Trivial information should have no bearing on the case. For instance, recounting the weather on a particular day has no bearing unless it directly relates to the patient's condition. In another example, you note that a patient presents in pajamas. Record this information only if it is significant. Otherwise it is just trivial information with no relevance to the case.

The report writer is striving to reduce verbiage and eliminate trivial and irrelevant information. He must also be aware of the flow of the remaining information. Organize the recorded data into logical groups. Thoroughly describe the mechanism of injury before proceeding to the effects of the mechanism on the patient. For example, describe how the automotive struck the tree at a high rate of speed. Tell what happened to the occupants at the point of impact. Then proceed to describe the effect of the mechanism of injury on the patient.

Use of Abbreviation. Any abbreviations used should be common abbreviations. (Refer to appendices E and F for examples.) Other health care providers must readily recognize them.

Avoid excessive use of abbreviations. An example of excessive use is strings of abbreviations. Abbreviating like this blurs the meaning. After a while, strings of abbreviations lose all sense. They become nothing more than a run-on of alphabet letters. See the example below.

```
23 y/o/W M c/o ABD pn x2 d ↑ dp insp/ palp.

A&Ox3 sknWD perl ⊖ JVD bs==/clr ? ↓ snd @ bs

hx ⊕ ABD x6m ⊖Ṟmed    NKA Ṟ ⊖Δ → ER
```

Finally, from a legal standpoint they should be standard abbreviations. This means that you can find the abbreviation in an accepted medical text. Making up one's own abbreviations creates confusing documents that are open to interpretation. A skillful attorney could easily turn the use of original (non-standard) abbreviations against the report writer in a court room. It raises a whole array of doubts and innuendo about the EMT or paramedic's knowledge and competency. You look inept because of the use of non-standard abbreviations. The report might never see a courtroom or deposition. Nevertheless, imagine other health care workers trying to figure out what you meant. Just because your abbreviations are clear to you, they will likely make no sense to others.

Some patients present with multiple complaints. It might be necessary in these cases to arrange the history of present illness under separate problem headings. This separation may be easier for both the report writer and any later readers.[27]

Be careful if and when you abbreviate. Use standard abbreviations, not ones you make up.

Past Medical History

This is where you record the illnesses that the patient has had in the past. They may or may not have anything to do with the present illness.

Write the *Past Medical History* (PMH), as well as later parts of the report, in a style different from the HPI. Writing these parts in complete sentences is not so important. Therefore, an economy of time and space should result. Consider the points already made about abbreviations as you write this section and the other sections of the report.

The PMH lists significant illnesses, injuries, surgical procedures, allergies, and medications. Here is where to report any lifestyle habits such as alcohol or tobacco use or drug abuse. Weigh the significance of any minor items mentioned by the patient. Are they pertinent to the case? If the report writer is not sure about the pertinence, then inclusion would be prudent. With experience, some items will obviously be significant. This may include such items as a history of seizures, diabetes, hypertension, cardio-respiratory problems, etc. What may be more subtle are allergies. If the patient states an allergy to *anything*, write it down. It may not be significant at first, but could become important as the case develops. For instance, all allergies are significant to a physician prescribing medications.

On the subject of allergies, it may also be useful to determine if the reaction is merely a side effect. For example, consider the patient experiencing chest pain. When asked if he is allergic to any medications, the patient states he has an allergy to nitroglycerine. Accepting the statement by the patient at face value, the provider would avoid using a therapy with potential for benefit. On the other hand, asking the patient about the details of the reaction could uncover that the allergy consists of headache development. This is a side effect of nitroglycerine. The patient has a misunderstanding about allergies vs. side effects. The patient does not develop anaphylaxis. Therefore, the provider can still consider nitroglycerine as a viable therapy.

Note any significant family or social history. For example, heredity is a risk factor in coronary artery disease.[28] The patient presenting with symptoms of this disease entity may be a high risk patient. Similarly, ethnic or cultural response to illness may have a bearing on the present situation of the patient. Educational and economic status may also be significant.[29]

Physical Examination

This is the hands-on examination of the patient. Use your eyes, ears, hands, and nose.

The *Physical Examination* (PE) should include observations about the general appearance of the patient and the level of consciousness. Conduct the examination in a head-to-toe manner with pertinent findings noted. A finding may be positive, such as noting rales in the congestive heart failure patient. It might also be negative, such as noting the lack of dependent edema in the same patient.

Recording of vital signs, and when they were taken, is also a part of the physical examination. Often times EMTs and paramedics will record the vital signs and leave out when they were taken. This includes the situation of multiple sets of signs.

Changes in vital signs show trends in the status of the patient. The trend could be indicating either improvement or deterioration of the patient's condition. Trends occur during time frames that may be rapid or slow. To properly chart these trends, it is essential to record the time. A further point on this is that incomplete reports imply incomplete care.

Treatment Given

This is where you describe what you did to help the patient. Include what you did to keep the illness or injury from getting worse.

The *Treatment Given* (Rx) section is where you record what you did for the patient. All procedures performed and treatments given should be in line with your local protocols and scope of practice. The caveat "If you didn't write it, you didn't do it!" is as fitting here as elsewhere in the report. Some systems employ a series of check-off boxes to show the type of care given. For some cases, this section may be complete enough to stand on its own. If it is not, include your treatment in the narrative portion. It is not enough to state that you gave oxygen. What apparatus did you use? What was the flow rate (Liters per minute)? What was the route of administration? Oxygen is a drug. As with any drug that you give, you must accurately record how you gave it.

The run report forms used in many advanced life support systems have separate space for advanced life support procedures. This space should always contain some notation. If you start an intravenous fluid line, record the time, location, fluid and rate of administration. Also note the amount infused during treatment by the paramedic.

If you administer medications, note the time, drug, dosage and administration route. If you defibrillate the patient, note the time and watt seconds (joules) administered. Attach a copy of the electrocardiogram made during the procedure to the report.

The same is true for intubation. Was it nasal or oral? What size tube?

Record procedures attempted but not accomplished. For instance, if a paramedic tried to start an I.V. but was unsuccessful, record it as such. Also, if a patient is combative and resists your efforts, record it. This shows that you acted in good faith and tried to give appropriate care. The only reason the patient did not actually receive the care was because the patient resisted. If you do not record instances such as this, it appears you did nothing.

Changes During Transport

This is where you note whatever changed or did not change during the trip to the hospital.

Changes During Transport records changes that occur during treatment. The changes may be an improvement in coloration and decrease in chest pain after oxygen administration. They may also be a decrease in the level of consciousness followed by seizure activity. Note whatever changes occur while the patient is under your care. The apparently insignificant changes you note in the field may provide the key to diagnosis further along in the health care system.

Part of the job of the EMT and paramedic is to make and record observations about their patients in the prehospital setting. They see the circumstances that surround the illness or injury. Reproducing these circumstances in the hospital is not possible. The EMS provider must be aware of his role in the delivery of health care. The vantage point of EMTs and paramedics is unique. They are the only healthcare professionals who see the patient in the environment where illness and injury occur, and then treat and transport the patient to the hospital.

Notes

E.M.S. TRAINING PROGRAM
PATIENT CARE REPORT FORM

Patient Name:

Address:

DOB: Tel. #:

Next of Kin:

Address:

Relationship: Tel. #:

Transported to: Transport Priority:

Miles from: To:

❑ No Transport
REASON:

Trip #:   Date:

M.R.#:   Day:

Dispatch To: For:

Dispatch Time: Arrival Time:

To Hospital: At Hospital:

Location at Dispatch:

Billing Information (circle):

    Medicare   Medicaid   BC/BS

    Indust. Acc.   Self   Other

Subscriber:

Policy #:

Physical Exam

Eye Opening	❑ Spontaneous ❑ To Pain ❑ To Voice ❑ None
Verbal Response	❑ Oriented ❑ Confused ❑ Inappropriate ❑ Incomprehensible ❑ None
Motor Response	❑ Obedience ❑ Purposeful ❑ Withdrawal ❑ Flexion ❑ Extension ❑ None
Skin Condition	❑ Normal ❑ Cool ❑ Hot ❑ Pale ❑ Flushed ❑ Cyanotic ❑ Diaphoretic

Vital Signs

❑ Unable to Obtain   ❑ Not attempted
REASON:

Time	BP	Pulse	Resp. Rate/Effort

Allergies: ❑ None
                    ❑ Unknown

Current Medications: ❑ None
                    ❑ Unknown

Brought with Pt.? ❑ Yes ❑ No

Suspected Diagnosis: ❑ Chronic ❑ Acute

❑ Major Trauma ❑ Acute Medical ❑ Cardiac Arrest ❑ Shock

❑ Minor Trauma ❑ Minor Medical ❑ Cardiac Disorder ❑ ETOH

❑ Soft Tissue Injury ❑ Burns ❑ Ortho ❑ OD/Poison

❑ Neuro ❑ Seizure ❑ Psych ❑ OB/GYN ❑ Neonate

Emergency Care: ❑ CPR ❑ Extricate ❑ Back/Neck Immobilize

❑ Bleed Control ❑ Bandage ❑ Splint ❑ Heat/Cold Applied

❑ O₂ Administration: _____ liters/minute via _____

Airway: ❑ Cleared ❑ Oral ❑ Nasal Size: _____ ❑ Suction

Intubate: ❑ Endotracheal ❑ Nasotracheal Size: _____

Assist Ventilation: Rate: _____ Method: _____

❑ ECG Monitor ❑ Rhythm Strip Attached

Transport Position:

Chief Complaint/History/Changes in Patient Status

Advanced Life Support

Time	/	Medication	/	Rate/Dose	/	Route
	/		/		/	
	/		/		/	
	/		/		/	
	/		/		/	
	/		/		/	
	/		/		/	
	/		/		/	

Total Fluid Infused: _____ mls

DEFIB: Time: _____ Time: _____ Time: _____ Time: _____

       Joules: ___ Joules: ___ Joules: ___ Joules: ___

Medical Control: ❑ Direct ❑ C-MED Channel _____

MD#_____ Hospital _____

Hospital Notified Enroute: _____ ❑ Yes ❑ No

                    ❑ C-MED ❑ Dispatcher

Other Response Units/Agencies:

Unit #	EMT/Paramedic Signatures:
	_____ # _____ _____ # _____ # _____

Section A. Contains information identifying the patient and the patient's next of kin.

Section B. Contains information identifying the significant facts about the response.

Section C. Contains information about the transport. Also records cases when the patient was not transported by ambulance.

Section D. Contains essential billing information.

Section E. Contains information about the patient's mental status and appearance.

Section F. Space for accurately recording vital signs.

Section G. Record allergies and current medications the patient takes

Section H. Record what you suspect to be the general problem(s)

Section I. Record aspects of the emergency care you gave. This includes airway management and oxygen therapy.

Section J. This is the narrative report. Use the SEMS format to keep it organized.

Section K. Record Advanced Life Support intervention here

Section L. Identify the medical control physician and provide information about hospital notification here. The physician also can sign the orders in this space.

Section M. Make a record of the other units and agencies who responded.

Section N. Record your unit response number (mobile unit identifier), identify yourself and sign the report.

Specific Instructions for the Sections of the Sample EMS Report

The report on the preceding two pages is a sample run report on which can be recorded all of the necessary information. Actual reports may, of course, differ in layout. The following instructions elaborate on each section marked on the form.

Section A.

In this section, record the name, address, date of birth (DOB) and telephone number of the patient. Also record the name of the next of kin with address and telephone number. State the relationship of this person to the patient.

The information you provide here helps identify the patient for hospital personnel, for your service's billing purposes, and it also has use for research projects. From a medical and legal standpoint it identifies the patient you treated.

Section B.

This group of information is the record of the response. Assign a number to each call you respond to for tracking purposes. If you also record the hospital's medical record number, the case and information can be cross-referenced.

Record the date and day of the week the response took place here. These two items provide an easy reference point and are also valuable for cross checking the response information.

Also record the dispatch address and nature of the call in this section. In addition to the medical-legal perspective, it provides information about how effectively your system performs call triage. Simply put, does the call you arrive at usually appear similar to the one described during dispatch?

Recording the times when events occur forms an essential part of health care and public safety.

There can be questions of liability, medical-legal issues, police investigation, etc., where the correctly noted time is vital information for reconscructing events.

This section is one of the many places on the report where you record the time. The dispatch, scene arrival, enroute to hospital and hospital arrival times tell a lot about your E.M.S. system.

For example, are your dispatch to arrival times consistent with current industry standard? If not, maybe you need more units or a different deployment plan. Maybe you need both. Recording the location of the response unit at the time of dispatch helps this process. Sometimes it helps explain why it took so long for the ambulance to arrive.

Section C.

Where you took the patient and the priority of the transport have a bearing on how your system works. It also shows how critically ill or injured you perceived your patient to be. Does your system have a point-of-entry plan? If it does, do you follow the plan? This information also helps check the plan and its effectiveness.

Recording the mileage is useful for billing purposes. It can also be important if anyone questions what went on during transport. Using the mileage and transport times can help discredit any accusations of improper action on the part of the EMS personnel.

If there is no transport, record the reason. Were you cancelled enroute? Were you unable to locate a valid incident when you arrived? Was it a police matter? Remember any situation where you arrive and evaluate patients requires more detailed documentation. This is particularly true of patient refusals.

Write a report.

Section D.

Getting the correct billing information helps you get paid. If you work for a private service, this is your bread and butter. If you work for a municipal service or authority, this is one way you can turn your service from a cost center to a profit center. If yours is one of the many volunteer services, successful billing may make the difference whether your neighbors receive any EMS service at all.

E.M.S. is expensive. People have insurance plans to pay for it. You are responsible for helping to get the billing information. Get as much of it as you can. The flip side of this is that ability to pay should never be a consideration in an emergency. Indeed, some states have specific laws and regulations prohibiting any consideration of ability to pay in a medical emergency.

Section E.

This section records level of consciousness using the trauma score. Use it to help you describe the level of consciousness. Research projects find this format useful as well.

The section also calls attention to skin condition, another valuable diagnostic sign. Combine the information in this section with the next one on vital signs. Notice you are focusing on many of the commonly used diagnostic signs. They tell you a lot about your patient.

Section F.

Record vital signs here. Write down the time they are taken. Take multiple sets of vital signs on critical patients, or during calls where you have the patient in your care for an extended time. If any or all of the vital signs were unobtainable, or there were circumstances where it was unwise to do so, make a note of it. Give a reason.

Some reasons might be a combative or agitated patient making it impossible to get an accurate set of signs. Perhaps you find yourself facing a hostile patient having a psychological emergency. If no threat to life exists, assess the situation a bit further. Trying to take vitals might make the situation worse. Consider using all of this to your advantage. You might be able to negotiate a peaceful transport. Finally, remember that a competent patient has the right to refuse treatment. This includes the taking of vital signs.

Section G.

This section provides space for recording allergies and current medications the patient takes. You may choose to include all of this information here or note it in the narrative. You also may choose to list it in both places. If you include it in the narrative only, make a note here telling that to the reader.

Section H.

This portion contains a series of check-off boxes where you indicate what you, as an EMT or paramedic, suspect to be the problem. It provides the reader with an idea of the problem at a glance. It is a useful tool for research and case review.

Section I.

This section is also a series of check-off boxes and has a few blanks to fill in. Record the care you gave the patient here. It is a concise statement of treatment. Expand on it in the narrative. It also contains precise information about airway management and oxygen therapy.

You also describe some advanced level interventions and the position you transported the patient in. The section has medical, legal, quality assurance and research applications. It is also useful to the people who do the billing in your organization.

Section J.

Section J is the narrative. Use the SEMS format here to describe what occurred on the call. Remember that what you write survives long after you leave the patient at the hospital. It follows the patient through the healthcare system. It follows cases through the court system, the medical examiner's office and E.M.S. administration. The narrative has a place in both quality control and training issues, as well as research. Write clearly and concisely.

Section K.

Record any advanced life support procedures you performed here. This may include I.V. starts, medications administration and defibrillation. The format is standard for healthcare. Remember, be as accurate and precise as possible.

The following two examples record the administration of thiamine and dextrose through an intravenous line to an unconscious diabetic.

Advanced Life Support			
Time	Medication	Rate/Dose	Route
1300	D5W	KVO	L Arm
1301	Thiamine	1mg	IV
1303	D50	1 amp	IV

Example 1

Example 2 is more precise as to I.V. type and placement. It gives the specific dosage of all the medications. Remember that writing *1 Amp* does not describe the dosage. For examples of this, compare the adult and pediatric dosage contained in *1 Amp* of dextrose or sodium bicarbonate ($NaHCO_3$).

Advanced Life Support			
Time	Medication	Rate/Dose	Route
1300	D5W	KVO	118g1"④AC
1301	Thiamine	1mg	IVP
1303	Dextrose	25g	IVP

Example 2

Section L.

Record your communication with the medical control physician and the receiving hospital here. It can also be the place where the physician signs for orders given to paramedics.

Section M.

This space is for recording other units and agencies who were on the call. Examples include other ambulances, police and fire departments, social service agencies, and the medical examiner's office. This is just a partial list. The possibilities are myriad.

Recording this information is important from a legal perspective. It could also be very important if the case involves infectious disease exposure.

Section N.

This is where you identify the response unit you were in and who you are. The writer of the report should sign it. Depending on local protocol, you might note other responding members without actually having them sign the report. In any event, make sure that you identify each EMS member present on the call.

Although many EMTS and paramedics view this from a legal perspective, remember that infectious disease control is vital to your health and that of your family. Knowing who came in contact with a patient carrying a contagious disease could be a matter of life or death.

Some Points to Remember When Completing a Written Report

1. Be sure to fill in all the spaces. Do not leave blanks. If information was unobtainable, write it that way. If it did not apply, make note of it as not applicable. This notation shows you considered it. Interpret blank spaces to mean that you left something out. Did you neglect to do something?

2. Organize your thoughts before writing. Have a clear idea about what you are going to put on paper. Use some sort of format to keep you organized and on track. The SEMS format will work well.

3. Be clear and as brief as possible. Document them on a few lines. Some cases are lengthy, and require much writing. Most cases are not that way. Use headings to highlight topic areas, such as Chief Complaint or History of Present Illness. Keep to the topic. Place patient statements together whenever possible. Do not spread them all over the page. Try to keep some sort of organization and continuity of thought.

4. Abbreviations are all right to use, but keep to standard abbreviations. Other health care professionals must understand them. Your personal shorthand may mean nothing to the person who reads your report a few hours after you write it.

5. Avoid repeating the same phrase over and over (ie., "pt. states..."). Count how many times you use a word like *patient* or *pt.*. If you are using it more than once or twice, you are probably overusing it. It could also be making your report more wordy than it need be.

6. If you do not know something to be fact, avoid stating it as such. If it has the appearance of fact, then state that "it appears...". If you use a term that is subject to interpretation, such as "exhibits bizarre behavior," describe the behavior. This is particularly true if you based actions on the exhibited behavior (or did not act because of a subjective interpretation).

7. When writing reports, and when rereading them, try to imagine yourself in two other positions as a report reader. One is that of another health care provider who reads your report hours (or days) after you have left. The other is to imagine yourself in a courtroom two years later. Read the report from the viewpoint of an attorney who is doing everything possible to discredit you and your care.

   In either case, how will it read? How will it sound? Will it read as a report written by a competent healthcare professional? Were you thorough in assessing the patient and giving appropriate care? Or will you present as an individual unskilled in assessment and slipshod with care? Will you sound like a skilled medical professional, or will you raise questions about your competency?

These points are not all-inclusive. They are a guide to help you understand the need for better documentation. Then documentation becomes something that is improved with practice.

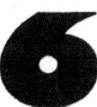

The Report as a Resource in the Hospital

The run report is a valuable resource for the hospital emergency department. It is more than just a way for EMTs and Paramedics to avoid litigation. Keep in mind the report benefits the patient as he journeys through the health care process.[30] The information in the trip sheet influences the care given by other providers. Proper documentation of the call gives the physician and nursing staff the insight and observations of the EMT/paramedic. That perspective is unique. No other member of the health care team sees the patient in the environment where the illness or injury occurred.

The documentation should be thorough. Some physicians consider certain points to be particularly important. These include mechanisms of injury and any environmental hazards that were present (such as toxic fumes). It also includes the proper recording of times. This means on scene times and when treatments were given. Record any medication that the patient currently takes, as well as the effect of any medication given in the field. Record vital signs before and after giving medications. Note any changes in patient condition affected by the care you give.

For example, assume you have a patient with chest pain and a history of angina. The man takes his prescribed nitroglycerine, but does not experience relief of pain as expected. You give him oxygen. Five minutes after receiving supplemental oxygen via nasal cannula at 4 liters per minute the patient is pain-free.

Remember to record all drug administration. Show the time, date, rate and route on the report.[31] (Remember that oxygen is a drug. Record its administration as you would any other drug.)

At times you will disagree with the doctor about the care to be given. You should, among other things, record any disagreement with the medical control physician about the care that you give. For example, you request a particular treatment that the medical control physician denies.[32] This difference of opinion prompts the case to be reviewed at a later time. It can be a positive learning experience for all concerned.

Also include changes that are consistent with protocol. For instance, the physician orders Atropine 1.0 mg I.V. for a patient experiencing symptomatic bradycardia. The paramedic gives Atropine 0.5 mg I.V. and the symptomatic bradycardia resolves.

If you are treating a cardiac patient, make a copy of the ECG. Label the strip. Include the patient's name, the date, and what leads are represented. Show the rhythm both before and after the prescribed care. Include a copy with the run report.[33]

The signature of the EMT/paramedic should be legible.[34] This is more than just for legal purposes. There is potential for future use of the run report to trace communicable diseases[35] and as part of research projects.

Realize that the run report is a valuable resource. It provides a unique view of the patient's condition. However, you must write it well. The well written report is a patient care tool. Hospital staff must read them. They need to become a part of the medical records. They need to be available for research. This is generally recognized practice in EMS systems.

In order for the report to be really useful, it has to be well-written.

EMTs and paramedics have a responsibility to document. The document must be clear and complete. Physicians and other providers have a responsibility to read the report.

The hospital and its medical staff have to view the EMS report as having important information about their patient.

The hospital has a responsibility to include the run report with the other medical records for the individual patient. Adverse results in the area of patient management can occur because of poor documentation by prehospital providers. It also can occur because the hospital staff ignores prehospital documentation.[36] A review by hospitals of the way they handle the prehospital medical record might help to remedy some of these cases.[37] The human cost is immense. Loss of life or permanent disability is a very real effect of the lack of diligence and attention to documentation.

7

Ambulance-to-Hospital
Radio Communication

Speaking to the hospital by radio intimidates some EMTs and paramedics. Normally secure individuals experience an increase in anxiety. They suddenly lose their ability to speak with authority. Instead, they speak in jumbled words and loose thought associations. The EMT/paramedic feels relief when the radio patch is over. Some hope that a large amount of time passes before having to call the hospital on the radio again.

Most formal EMT and paramedic instruction lacks definitive training, including practice sessions, in ambulance-to-hospital radio communications. Prehospital care providers find themselves left to figure out how to communicate with the hospital on their own. If they have a good role model, it will work out well. However, if the role model is a poor or non-existent one, expect a poor outcome.

Most EMTs and paramedics approach the use of the ambulance-to-hospital radio with good intentions. Many also need to approach the ambulance-to-hospital radio with a good plan. A good plan starts with planning ahead.

Develop a working knowledge of the triage systems and capabilities of the hospitals to which you usually transport. Speak with the emergency department staff. When you call them on the radio, what do they need to know? Equally important, what do they *not* need to know? Use radio time

Know what is important to say over the radio. Know what can wait until you can say it in person.

It is important that the hospital and prehospital personnel understand and cooperate with each other.

efficiently. The emergency department staff also needs to know what information the EMTs and paramedics consider important. Both sides need to understand each other.

The days of letting the hospital know of every transport are over. At least they are in most urban and suburban systems. That amount of radio traffic would overwhelm the staff of both the communications centers and the emergency departments. EMTs and paramedics need to know which cases require a hospital notification. This means prioritizing transports according to severity when deciding when to call the hospital.

A simple set of questions can help with the decision:

1. Is the illness or injury life-threatening?

2. Do additional staff and resources need to be mobilized before the arrival of the patient?

If the answer is yes to any of these questions, then call. If it is not, forego notification in most cases.

The EMT/paramedic needs to know that prompt triage and treatment of the critical patient awaits at the hospital. The needs of the emergency department are usually straightforward. A few beds exist for critical patients. A few staff personnel (physician, nurse, technical and support staff) are present. These limited resources need effective use. Medical patients need different resources than surgical patients. Proper assignment of resources is necessary.

The goal is to provide better care for all patients.

Proper notification enhances delivery of these services. It gives the hospitals a few minutes to move patients around so they can make room for the newly arriving critical patient. They can assemble the necessary medical or surgical staff. It also gives them a few moments to think about the case before the arrival of the patient. An efficient transfer of patient and information takes place and the patient receives better service.

So what should the EMT/paramedic say on the radio? When speaking to the triage person, give that individual enough information to decide what to do. The person doing triage needs to know essentials. Is the case medical or surgical? How sick is the patient? Are special services necessary?

The EMT/paramedic needs to organize the notification. Many places refer to the ambulance-to-hospital notification as a *radio patch*. Organize it the same way that you organize written reports—use the SEMS format. Describe the patient characteristics. Give the age and gender of the patient. State the chief complaint. Give a *brief* outline of the history. Here you give only enough information to help the listener understand the problem. State major findings from the physical exam. Here again, you only need to state the findings that effect triage. Tell the hospital what you have done for the patient. Include a statement about how the patient responds to the care you are giving.

Accomplish this quickly. If you are speaking for more than 30 to 60 seconds, you are speaking too long. Remember, the purpose is to help the hospital prepare for and triage the patient.

For example, consider a patient with a gunshot wound to the chest. The patient needs surgery. The operating room needs alerting. What does triage need to know?

Tell triage the age of the patient, the location of the wound, level of consciousness and the vital signs. Include breath sounds. State in a couple of phrases the care you are giving. Give an estimate of how long it will take you to arrive at the hospital. Remember, be brief and to the point.

For another example, consider the patient with chest pain, presumed to be cardiac in origin. In this case, the hospital will need to provide a bed with a

Organize your thoughts before you press the button.

Keep it brief!

monitor, examine the patient and develop a treatment plan.

Tell triage the age and gender of the patient. Briefly describe the pain and how it began. If the patient has a significant history, state it. Give the vital signs. State the major physical findings. Is the patient alert and oriented? Skin warm and dry or cool and moist? Is the patient breathing well? Does the patient take medication?

If you are a paramedic state what you find on the monitor. Then state what you are doing for the patient. Tell the hospital if your treatment has any effect. Give an estimate of how long it will take you to arrive at the hospital. Remember to be brief and to the point.

A medical patient notification will probably take longer than one for the trauma patient. Keep it under a minute in length. Ideally, try to do it in about 30 seconds. The person on the other end of the radio needs to know enough to help them decide where to place the patient. He is not deciding about the treatment the patient actually gets in the emergency department.

You will probably have much more information about the patient than you can present in this setting. It is all important information. Save it for when you are face-to-face with the physician and staff. Tell it to those who will be doing the actual patient care. The doctor and nurse need to know all the fine points of information you have to offer about the case. Triage does not.

Speaking with Medical Control

The field paramedic is the eyes, ears, and hands of the medical control physician. This role of physician extender creates a bond and trust that is unique in healthcare. The medical community places only a few healthcare occupations in this role.

Emergency medical technicians operate in a like manner. They are also accountable to the medical community. EMTs should keep in mind there are times when they will need to speak with the medical control physician.

Effective radio communication skills are essential for the prehospital care provider. An understanding of the communication medium must be borne in mind when speaking on the radio. Remember that you are the eyes, ears, and hands of the physician. The physician is relying on you to make an accurate assessment of the patient and the situation and environment in which the patient presents. The orders that you receive (or do not receive) are based on this.

Remember that you are the eyes, ears, and hands of the physician.

At times, you will expect a certain set of orders, but a different set will be given. When this happens, you must ask yourself if you presented the case properly. You might have presented it very well, and the physician has picked up on a subtle part of the presentation. Enhanced patient care is the result.

On the other hand, you may have given a poor presentation. You gave the physician the wrong impression and the orders are not in line with the best patient care. It also might be that the physician withholds orders because he cannot get a grasp of the situation from your report. When these situations occur, you will have to clarify the situation and see if the medical control physician wishes to change the treatment plan.

The prehospital practitioner must learn to paint an accurate picture using words alone. The physician cannot see, hear, or touch the patient. The EMT or paramedic needs to keep this in mind. You have to convey your clinical observations and impressions to the medical control physician solely by your voice. The words you choose and voice inflections convey a message. Be aware of the message you are sending.

Your words must paint a clear picture. Choose them well.

You also need to give a thorough and detailed description of the current patient condition and the events leading up to it. The SEMS format presented in this manual will help you with this description. You will still need to give a description that includes your impressions gained from the senses of sight, sound, touch and smell. Remember, you are the extension of the physician. You have to be his eyes, ears, and hands.

For example, if you are reporting on a respiratory patient, your findings as to skin coloration, diaphoresis, respiratory rate and effort, patient position, use of accessory muscles, and lung sounds will all have to be included. This information will need organization. Blend it together with the other information you obtain about the patient. Then tell the story. Remember to paint the picture in the mind of the physician. If you find that the orders you want do not come through consistently, you need to consider improving your skills as an artist. You may need more practice at "painting the picture" over the radio.

Another clue to self-assessment of your radio communication skills is to listen to the questions the physician asks after you give your report. Are you always asked to get more information? If so, are you consistently missing the same points? If the answer is yes to these questions, the medical control physicians are telling you ways to improve your performance. Act on it!

Another way of improving is to analyze what you said. Put yourself in the position of the medical control physician. Did you convey the message clearly? If you were on the other end of the radio, would you have understood what was going on in the field? Also, ask the physician what his impression was. Look for ways to improve. Start with yourself. Good communication skills are the result of practice. Always try to improve.

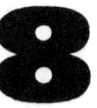

Presenting the Case in the Emergency Department

When you present the case in the emergency department, use the SEMS format. It is the same one that you will use when you write the report. Make sure you have the attention of the staff. Be assertive and descriptive. Point to physical findings. Make sure that they understand the case you are presenting. Ask for questions after you are done. In this way you will present yourself and the patient in a professional manner.

In the emergency department you will probably have to give at least two reports. One report will be given to the person who does triage. In many hospitals this is a nursing role. A second report will be given to the emergency department staff who will be treating the patient.

The report to the triage person does not need details. The SEMS format is still useful, but give an abbreviated version. Remember that triage is sorting. The person doing triage needs enough information to decide where in the emergency department to assign the patient. The seriousness of the illness or injury will have a bearing on this, as will the type of illness or injury.

Triage needs enough information to sort the patient to the right bed assignment.

Many hospitals divide their emergency department into areas for acute and non-acute patients. Patients with sudden, severe onset of symptoms or critical injuries can expect assignment to an acute care area. Patients who have illnesses of a more chronic nature without an acute exacerbation, or minor illnesses and injuries, receive an assignment to a non-acute area.

The EMT or paramedic should be aware that such systems exist. If you are routinely transporting to the same hospital or hospitals, you should become familiar with the triage process at the hospitals you serve. This will help you to take pertinent information from the case and report it to triage. You will waste much less time by not talking about case aspects that have no bearing on triage.

After the triage person has heard your report, listen to the questions asked of you. If you find that the questions usually center on minor clarifications, then you are probably giving a good report.

Remember, how you react to triage, and how triage reacts to you, affects the patient.

However, if the triage person consistently asks you for more detailed information after your report, you probably need to work on your reporting skills. You also may find that the triage person ignores you and goes right to the patient either before or after your report. If you or your company or department has a history of poor care, poor reporting skills, or both, you can expect this response.

On the other hand, the triage person may need some education about the role and function of prehospital healthcare. It might be worthwhile to sit down with the emergency department personnel who do triage and find out what it is that they expect from you. What information helps them decide where to assign the patient? What information means little at triage and just serves to slow down the process? Find out what you need to do. Then do it. It is also possible to earn respect by presenting yourself as a competent, knowledgeable, professional health care giver.

Triage and prehospital EMS must understand each other's needs and capabilities.

The SEMS format will help you give the report. The format will help keep you on track and organized. You will properly and professionally present the patient and yourself. An emphatic point is that you need to have the attention of your audience. If possible, wait until the treatment team assembles.

The second report you give in the hospital is to the staff who will be treating the patient. This includes physicians, physician assistants, nurses, nurses aides, respiratory therapists, and others. These individuals share an interest in the patient, although the information they need from you may vary with their function in the emergency department. If you give a clear, detailed but concise report, you can expect that your report will be informative, useful, and well-received. People will pay attention to your report.

The goal here is to give a complete report once. You should not have to start, stop, and start again as more team members arrive. This results in a disorganized report. It is difficult for the rest of the team to follow, and frustrating for you. Once you are into the report, do not allow interruptions. Politely but firmly inform late arrivals that you will continue the report and then answer questions after the report is complete. Do your job competently and professionally. You will find that most emergency department personnel will afford you this courtesy. They will also be on time for the next patient report that you give.

In some cases of minor illnesses or injuries it is proper to give the report only to the nurse who will care for the patient, since the physician may not see the patient for a while. The report must be complete and properly delivered. Remember—this is another opportunity to build respect and confidence in your capabilities. It also helps build respect for and confidence in the EMS industry, in general.

In critical cases, the emergency department personnel need to gain a lot of knowledge about the patient in a short span of time. They may never have seen this patient before. You, however, have already spent time with the patient. In most cases you should have much information to give. Prepare to give it.

Sometimes, for reasons beyond your control, you will not have much information to give. Do not be afraid to acknowledge that you do not have all of the information. "I don't know" is the right answer in this case. Never present your opinion as fact. If you have an opinion, state it as such at a proper time. Your opinion may be well formed and useful. Remember to present it as opinion, not fact.

If you find that you are saying "I don't know" a lot with a variety of different patients, then you probably need to work on your interview and history taking skills. Pay attention to the questions asked in the hospital. Much of the information that the emergency department gathers is easy to gather in the field. It only requires the development of good history-taking skills.

When you are asking questions and gathering information in the field, use the SEMS format. It will help you gather the information in an organized way. It also will help you sort it out. Then you can present it to the emergency department personnel in an organized and efficient manner.

Get their attention. Then give a report that is organized and thorough. Remember to keep it as short and to the point as possible.

In some cases, this will be easy. You will already have notified the hospital by radio before arriving with a critically ill or injured patient. Everyone is waiting for you. At other times, the patient will not be so sick, and you will not have notified the hospital ahead of time. In cases such as this, wait until the team assembles. While waiting, you can move the patient to the hospital bed as you ask about the expected arrival of absent team members. If possible, make sure the person who will be running the case is present.

Emergency department nurses perform many vital roles in the EMS system. Developing a good rapport with them and enabling them to develop one with you benefits all concerned. The patient is the ultimate benificiary.

Special Reporting Situations

Consent

You must get consent before treating a patient. The patient may imply consent by conduct. The patient can provide consent either orally or in writing. Consent must be informed in order to be valid or effective consent.[38] EMTs and paramedics can make errors and misjudgments about the issue of informed consent. *Informed* means that the person clearly understood the choices offered to them.[39] If the person does not understand, the person cannot consent. If it was a family member or friend or passer-by who called for the ambulance, make sure you obtain the person's consent before treating and transporting him. (Refer to Appendix D for definitions of types of consent.)

People summon an ambulance to help them in time of medical emergency. They are ready to consent to reasonable care and transportation. This is why they called the ambulance. Nevertheless, it is still good practice to explain even the simplest of procedures to the patient. For instance, inform them that you are going to take their blood pressure. Involve the patient in the process. Tell them this is standard practice and that you pass on the information to the hospital. It all helps to give patients the proper care for their illness or injury. This type of involvement requires the EMT or paramedic to treat the patient as a person, not just another case.

The patient must agree to the treatment.

With regard to invasive therapies, inform patients when you are starting I.V.s. Ask them if they have ever had an I.V. before. Tell them when you are giving medications. Give a brief explanation of what you are about to do.

Tell them the type of medication. Explain in simple terms what you expect the medication to do. This includes giving the drug oxygen to the patient.

Try to help the patient understand how what you are doing helps him.

Inform the patient of any possible side effects. An example is developing a headache after taking nitroglycerine. Weave consent into the development of patient histories. While eliciting the history, ask questions about allergies and medications. Evolve this into the proposed treatment of the present condition. This can help assure informed consent. It links the current situation to a previous situation. If he is unsure about the current situation, this can help resolve anxiety. The patient will develop a familiarity with the present situation.

Talk to the patient. Let the patient know what is going on.

Advise the patient that you are in contact with the physician at the hospital. Explain how you are talking to the doctor by radio (if this is the case). Let him know that you are working under the doctor's direction. Explain that the physician has ordered the I.V. Explain that the doctor is prescribing the medication. Tell the patient you are giving the medication. This helps to make clear the role of the paramedic as a physician extender. It may also allay fears about what is occurring, and gain the cooperation of some marginally cooperative individuals.

Remember that competent patients always have the right to change their minds and withdraw consent. When this situation occurs, clearly document it. Make it very clear that it is an informed withdrawal of consent. Make the patient aware of the implications of withdrawing consent. Explain this in words he understands. For instance, not taking the medication could make the condition worse. If it is a trauma patient, explain why you need to immobilize them. Explain they could suffer permanent disability if a spinal injury exists. Tell

The competent patient has the right to withdraw consent. Make sure he or she understands what is being done.

them this is why you are placing them on a spineboard.

Patient Refusals

Is the patient oriented to person, place, and time?

Does the patient understand who you are, why you are there, and what could happen as a result of the refusal?

You are responsible. Do you feel comfortable letting the patient refuse treatment?

Any competent person has the right to refuse medical treatment. On the face value of this statement, it might appear easy to deal with a refusal. After all, if they say they do not want to go to the hospital, that is all you need. And if there is any doubt, get the answers to a few questions. Assuming these patients are conscious, do they know who and where they are? Do they know the day and the date? An oriented person knows all of this and answers the questions appropriately.

Is the refusal informed? If they understand and acknowledge the implications of the refusal, then the answer is yes. If the patient does not comprehend the implications of the refusal, the answer is no. No informed refusal exists. Therefore, the refusal is not valid.

Answer another question as well. Is the patient mentally competent? Only a mentally competent person can refuse treatment.[40,41] An intoxicated person cannot. Do you suspect intoxication? Is the patient under the influence of drugs? Does the patient have a head injury? These patients are not competent to refuse. The suicidal patient may well know the answer to who and where they are, and what the day and date are. Nevertheless, the patient is not competent to refuse.

This is the dilemma for the EMT or paramedic. To complicate matters, other public safety agencies may accept the refusal. However, are you satisfied that the person has refused? The case could become the subject of a legal proceeding. The EMT or paramedic must bear in mind they are the medically trained person on scene.[42] Members of the other agencies will be quick to point out how they were not responsible. They were not the medically

Erring on the side of providing care is better than omitting care.

trained person on scene. They called the ambulance. That was their responsibility.

The EMT/paramedic must decide. Is it an informed refusal? An acceptable refusal is one made by a competent patient who understands the implications of the refusal. If there is doubt, remember that erring on the side of providing care is better than omitting care. Omitting care can cause problems later.

Remember, how you document a patient refusal is important. This documentation can have an impact in the future. Questions about the judgment of the EMT/paramedic will arise. In addition to documenting the case for the present, the report writer must always look to the future. How will today's report sound to an impartial group of people in the future? Did the EMT/paramedic act in good faith? Did the EMT/paramedic act in the best interest of the patient? Did the EMT/paramedic act to protect the patient's rights?

Ask questions from the opposite point of view as well. Was the EMT/paramedic cold and detached, without empathy for the patient? Will a lack of concern show through? Did the health care provider assure the patient understood the implications of the refusal? Was the refusal informed? Was the patient competent? In the real world of EMS, there often are no easy answers to these questions.

You must write reports that impart a sense of the present circumstances to some unknown reader in the future. The documentation should clearly relate the events that took place. It should provide an accurate description of what people said and did before the patient's decision to refuse treatment and transport. The EMT/paramedic accepted the refusal as informed and competent. What was that decision based upon? The decision must be shown to have been sound.

Considering the previous discussion, simply writing *pt. refusal* on the trip sheet is not enough. It has no place in a system that requires accurate

The patient you do not transport today could cost you time, money, and worry tomorrow.

It is essential to develop the skill of documenting the non-transport situation.

documentation. The EMT/paramedic who sees fit to document in such a manner is just looking for trouble. This manner of documenting implies poor patient care and may show incompetence. Nothing was done. Who was the patient? Did the patient understand the implications of the refusal? It does not take too much imagination to picture the bereaved family saying "the ambulance came and did nothing." A review of the record shows they are right. They wrote nothing. Nothing was done. Case closed. The poorly documented refusal invites an adverse judgment against the EMT/paramedic and the employer of the unskilled report writer.

It is urgent that EMTs and paramedics master the art of effective report writing. No area is more critical for the development of this skill than the area of the non-transport situation. Dispatchers send ambulances to transport people to the hospital. When transportation does not occur, record the reasons. The call to service and the service response implies a contract. A breached contract is one not brought to completion. Litigation may follow if a party claims that a breach in contract has occurred.

What should you document? Record the day, date and appropriate times. Record the address where the dispatcher sent the ambulance. Get patient's name, address, date of birth and any other information such as telephone number and next of kin. Record the vital signs and mental status of the patient.

Note that you advised the patient of the extent of the illness or injury. Show that you described to the patient the likely course of events if the illness or injury went untreated. Record that the patient acknowledged what you said. Document that the patient understood the implications of what you said. Note any treatments attempted by you. Also note if the patient resisted your efforts to help.

Write down the names and addresses of witnesses. The patient should *clearly* sign a statement stating you told them what could happen if they refuse treatment. Note the refusal is by their own free choice. Having the refusal *clearly* signed is very important. The hastily scrawled signature obtained by many EMTs and paramedics usually bears little resemblance to the patient's actual signature. Later, an attorney can easily show that a dissimilarity exists. This will support the argument that the patient was under stress. The patient could not competently refuse. The plaintiff was so emotionally distraught by the incident that he could not even sign a piece of paper properly.[43]

Modify this for the belligerent patient who refuses treatment and transportation. A patient like this may refuse to even discuss the situation with the EMT/paramedic. Getting a clear and legible signature on a piece of paper is out of the question. Here the report writer should document the efforts to get an informed refusal. Discussions and on-scene times may be very important here.

Use your report to record the effort to reason with the patient. Use this, coupled with documentation of a lengthy on-scene time, to show that the EMT/paramedic acted in good faith, and used all reasonable means that were available to provide care and transportation to the patient. If you think the patient is making a poor judgment by refusing, consider using the influence of family members and significant others to get the patient to agree to go to the hospital. If you think the patient should go to the hospital, be persistent. If you are going to make a mistake, make it on the side of providing good patient care.

Some patients will be uncooperative. They may be competent and are fully within their rights to refuse. You are responsible for documenting the events occurring on the call. If there is a reasonable doubt as to competency, then consider discussion with the proper law enforcement agency. This situation also indicates a need to discuss the occurrence with the medical director of the service. The on-line medical director is a valuable resource in cases such as this.

Child Abuse

Lack of reasonable care and protection.

Child abuse and neglect has been a topic of discussion for centuries. The traditional view saw child abuse as a private family problem. It is a fairly recent area of involvement for health care workers.[44]

The federal Child Abuse Prevention and Treatment Act (Public Law 93-247) provides a definition. It is "...the physical or mental injury, sexual abuse, negligent treatment or maltreatment of a child under the age of eighteen by a person who is responsible for the child's welfare under circumstances which indicate that the child's health or welfare is harmed."[45]

In Massachusetts, Chapter 119 of the General Laws, Sections 51A through 51F concerns the subject of child abuse. Most states have similar statutes in existence.[46] EMS personnel working in states other than Massachusetts should check the wording of the statute in their particular state.

Section 51A deals with mandated reporters. The term *mandated reporter* means someone who legally must report suspected cases of child abuse. The statute lists various professional occupations as mandated reporters. The list includes emergency medical technicians. The statute provides in pertinent part as follows:

> ...who in his or her professional capacity shall have reasonable cause to believe that a child under the age of eighteen is suffering serious physical or emotional injury resulting from abuse inflicted upon him or her... shall immediately report such condition to the Department by oral communication and by making a written report within 48 hours after such oral communication.[47]

Consider the requirement for EMTs and paramedics to report suspected cases of abuse and neglect. When considering this, the question of what constitutes abuse or neglect bears some discussion.

We all have violent impulses. In theory, anyone is a potential child abuser, but most people can control these violent impulses. Abusive persons cannot. Certain characteristics of abusive families that have emerged. They are:

1. an unfulfilled need to be nurtured and dependent

2. fear of relationships

3. inability to care for or protect a child

4. lack of nurturing, child-rearing practices (including unrealistic expectations of a child's developmental abilities)

5. lack of support systems

6. marital problems

7. life crises[48]

Abusers may have any of the characteristics, although it is neither common nor necessary that they have all of them.

The prehospital health care provider should be aware of the physical and behavioral indicators of child abuse. As an EMT/paramedic, you must identify those characteristics. You need to distinguish them from normal physical findings and normal developmental stages in the child patient.

Divide physical indicators into the following general groupings:

1. Bruises and welts. Where on the body are the bruises located? Are there bruises in various stages of healing? Do they exhibit patterns (Does it look like an object struck the child)? Is there evidence of repeated beatings?

The abuser could be anyone. Abuse is not tied to ethnic groups or economic status.

Learning about child development will help you sort out the bumps and bruises.

2. Burns. Is there evidence that a child has had body parts immersed in hot liquid? Are there cigarette burns? Has the child been bound? Do you see rope burns?

3. Lacerations and abrasions. Pay particular attention to lacerations and abrasions found on infants. Also pay attention to such injuries found on the external genitalia.

4. Skeletal injuries. Where is the fracture and is the story about the injury consistent with the physical findings?

5. Head injuries. Includes evidence of hair pulling as well as blunt trauma and injuries that would result from shaking. (Look for findings that suggest subdural hematomas and retinal hemorrhage or detachment.)

6. Internal injuries that result from blunt trauma to the abdomen.[49]

Consider in all this whether the story of what happened (the mechanism of injury) is consistent with the injury. Consider whether it is consistent with the capability of the child at its present stage of development.[50] (Ask yourself if the child can perform or take part in the activity that allegedly caused the injury.)

The behavioral indicators are the exhibition of the coping mechanisms the child has developed to survive in the abusive environment. For instance, does the child appear passive? Is the exhibited behavior designed to maintain a low profile even in the face of obviously painful injuries? Conversely, does the child engage in activity that is aggressive to call attention to himself?[51]

What is the relationship of parent and child? Is there a role reversal or does the child appear dependent on the parent? Is the child's development lagging in relationship to its peer group?[52]

Look at how the parent behaves. Does the parent act overly concerned and protective about the child? This may indicate the the parent is afraid of what the child will say if left alone. The opposite response, lack of concern, should create concern on the part of the EMT/paramedic.

The EMT/paramedic should become knowledgeable about child abuse. EMTs and paramedics need to attain an understanding of the underlying family dynamics. The acquisition of this type of knowledge will result in an increased awareness of, and sensitivity to, the potential abuse situation.

Neglect is another form of abuse. It is lack of reasonable care and protection of the child by the caretaker. The lack of reasonable care may take the form of lack of supervision, inadequate clothing, or poor hygiene. It also is lack of medical or dental care, poor nutrition or inadequate shelter.[53]

The reporter should understand that he may not agree with a specific child-rearing practice or cultural value. Your subjective values do not define abuse. Rate the situations for reasonable care and protection. Also, poverty and neglect are two entities. Being poor does not mean that you neglect your children. For instance, consider a particular family unit in a lower socioeconomic group. Just because they are in a lower socioeconomic group does not mean they abuse children. The root of child abuse and neglect is in psychological elements, not economics. These elements make the abusers unable to cope with personal and environmental factors in their lives. Grasp the size of the problem. Consider the following statistical compilations and what they show:

The Department of Health and Human Services completed a study in 1980. The study determined abuse or neglect occurs to 652,000 children in the United States each year.[54] In 1984 that figure had risen to 727,000.[55] That same year, Massachusetts reported 41,116 cases. The state substantiated 14,556 of these.[56] In 1986, Massachusetts reported 49,799 cases of which the state substantiated 18,295.[57] For the year 1985, the breakdown of the reports by type (49,465 reported, 17,830 substantiated) in Massachusetts showed neglect in 52%. The rest of the breakdown showed abuse in 34% and sexual abuse in 14%.[58]

One half of all reported cases concern neglect, while the other half takes the form of physical abuse. Also, the numbers of reports and substantiated cases have risen steadily through the 1980s.

It is possible that abuse is on the rise. It is also possible that the start of data collection coupled with many mandated reporters have brought to the surface the size of the problem. If the national experience mirrors the experience in Massachusetts, expect the rate of increase to taper off. Annual percentage increases will stabilize in the single digits.[59]

The Reporting Procedure in Massachusetts

Reporters make initial notification over the telephone. The Child-At-Risk Hotline maintains a toll-free telephone number 24 hours per day (1-800-792-5200). As a reporter, you make an oral report including the name, address and estimated age of the child. You also report the names and addresses of the parent or caretaker. Know what language is spoken by the child and the caretaker. They will ask your name, address, telephone number and professional relationship with the child. (Nonmandated reporters may request to remain anonymous.)

They will ask the nature of the present and, if indicated, prior abuse, neglect or injury. You also will need to assess the level of risk of further harm, and determine if that risk is imminent. You also will describe the circumstances under which the situation first came to your attention. For the EMT/paramedic, this circumstance is usually during one's professional occupation. As a health care provider, you respond to medical emergencies in the community. Additionally, report any action taken by you to treat, shelter or help the child. You must submit a report in writing within 48 hours.[60]

It makes sense to fill out the written report right away. Then, refer to the written report when you make the oral report. This will keep you organized. It will also keep the information consistent.

The Department of Social Services provides a report form. They refer to this as a 51A. The law requires all mandated reporters to file a 51A in cases of suspected abuse within 48 hours. Timeliness is an issue. Mandated reporters may be penalized for their failure to report.[61]

Confusion exists about the responsibility to file if multiple mandated reporters deal with the case. This is a common occurrence in the emergency medical setting. The EMT/paramedic sees the patient. They transport to the hospital and the hospital staff (physicians, nurses, etc.) sees the child. Many mandated reporters become involved. The question then arises as to who files the report. The EMT and the paramedic must file their own report. Though the physician and the hospital are filing reports, this does not relieve the EMT or paramedic from their responsibility. Nor does it relieve the hospital and its staff from their responsibility to file because the EMT/paramedic is filing. The law clearly states that all mandated reporters must file.[62]

Other issues that surface during the reporting process are those concerning accuracy. If something is a known fact, state it as such. If it represents a hypothesis on the part of the EMT/paramedic, state that it is a guess. This is not to dissuade reporters from providing their subjective assessment of the situation. It is to help the investigator determine the reliability of information.

EMTs and paramedics work night and weekend shifts as well as day shifts. Because of this it is helpful to say when you are available. This also helps if the investigator needs to contact them.[63]

As a final note, if other children were present but uninjured, report it. Note that you saw them at the time of the incident. By noting the uninjured children who were also present, you answer the question about the immediate well-being of the other children.[64] This alleviates any anxiety about them. It also saves the time of the investigator for use in dealing with the case. The investigator need not spend time seeking to check the status of the other children present at the reported incident. It also gives the report completeness.

Elder Abuse

At the opposite end of the life cycle, the elder members of the community may also be the targets of abuse. This abuse takes the form of physical abuse, emotional abuse or neglect. Child abuse captures the attention of the media and the populace. Elder abuse may be no less of a problem that faces our society as we enter the twenty-first century. A phenomenon of modern society is that our rapidly expanding technology, particularly medical technology, has increased the human life span, especially in the western world. As a result of this, disease processes that once were terminal are now treatable. The members of our society are living longer.

The younger members of the community increasingly find themselves in the position of caretaker for the elderly. This occurs in a youth oriented society. Having to deal with a growing child can create stresses which some people are unable to cope with. Having to deal with elderly family members who may be a burden in their later years can also be stressful.

Apply much of that said about child abuse to the elderly. The signs of physical abuse are remarkably similar. Look for other types of abuse. Is the elder person passive or anxious? Is the elder showing changes in behavior while the caregiver is present? Is the care given to the elder consistent with the apparent assets? Do you sense there is more financial ability to care for the elder than you are seeing?[65]

Also view the financial situation from the perspective of self-abuse. Is the elder neglecting himself? The elder may live far away from relatives. Has the family abandoned the elder person?[66]

If you suspect elder abuse, look for hints such as frequent doctor visits that could be a cover-up for abuse. Other hints are delays in seeking help, injuries in various stages of healing and stories that do not match the injury or illness. Further hints include a poor interaction between the elder and the caregiver, and the elder not wanting to speak for himself, particularly while the caregiver is around.[67]

In Massachusetts, add EMTs and paramedics to the list of mandated reporters of cases of suspected elder abuse.[68] Similar information and reporting requirements apply in both cases. As a mandated reporter you also must file a report in writing. File this within 48 hours of the oral report.

Massachusetts defines elder abuse itself under M.G.L. Chapter 19A, Section 14-26. The Executive Office of Elder Affairs maintains an Elder Abuse Hotline (1-800-922-2275). Protective Services Workers assess the reported situations for potential abuse. Upon confirming abuse, they arrange for provision of services. The design of the services is to end or lessen abuse.[69]

The elderly population is a large consumer group of emergency medical services. The EMT/paramedic should be aware that the elderly do have rights. There are means of safeguarding those rights. Massachusetts legally protects from abuse and neglect any person over age 60 living in the community. Prehospital health care workers should be sensitive to this issue.

Crime Scene Management

The crime scene contains valuable evidence. It is also very fragile. Treat it with respect. You will find that the investigators will treat you with respect as well.

The crime scene is a fragile environment. It is a deteriorating piece of evidence. Each person who enters the crime scene needs to understand this and act responsibly.

EMS personnel must respond to crime scenes as part of their job. Interaction with law enforcement personnel is a daily occurrence. A crime scene response is an opportunity for building a solid rapport with other public safety personnel.

The following is a discussion of the duties and concerns of law enforcement personnel. It will help EMTs and paramedics to better understand the crime scene. It will show how the work that they do at a crime scene can help or hinder an investigation.

The responding police officer has many concerns. The first concern is to secure the scene. Subjects may still be present who pose a threat to the officer. They could also be a threat to other personnel (such as EMS) who are responding to the scene. Additionally, the officer does not want to become a casualty. He will be taking steps to secure the area.

The next concern of law enforcement personnel is to care for injured persons. The preservation of life takes precedence over the preservation of evidence. Here, a timely and efficient response by EMS can relieve the officer of this responsibility. It frees him to concentrate on accomplishing police matters (and there are many). They can also preserve more evidence.

After initial scene security and care for injured persons, the officer must identify witnesses and subjects, maintain control of the area, and set up contact with headquarters. They also must prepare notes to document actions and observations for later use.[70]

The roles of the police officer and the EMT/paramedic are complementary. The officer and the EMT/paramedic are both concerned with public safety. It is the perspective or viewpoint that is different. The officer has a responsibility to protect as much of the scene as possible. The question then is one of how the police officer and the EMT/paramedic can function together in this environment. The goal is a minimal hindrance of police work while still providing the best care for patients.

The place to begin thinking about this is not at the crime scene. It is in training programs and informational seminars. Each participant should have some clear ideas about his own role at the scene of a crime.

The police officer needs to know and understand that giving aid is a legitimate function of EMS. The role of the police officer is to aid and support that function.

The EMT/paramedic needs to know and understand that protecting evidence and later solving the crime is a legitimate police function. EMS personnel can help with this function without compromising their own role as health care providers.

The crime scene is dynamic. It attracts a diverse group of people.

To accomplish this adequately, the EMT/paramedic needs an understanding of the scene and the legal process. First, the scene is not a static, motionless place. It is dynamic. The crime scene has many people attracted to it. This includes law enforcement and EMS, and may include fire suppression personnel. Family members and acquaintances of the victim may also be present, as well as the news media. Many bystanders also may gather. In this diverse group of individuals there also may be witnesses and suspects.[71,72]

Anyone who enters the crime scene can be called into court. The EMT/paramedic will be called in along with his or her written report for all the world to see. Write it well.

The court can issue a summons to any person who is present at a crime scene. This includes officers. Any persons issued a summons must appear to testify as to their actions and observations at the crime scene.[73] The greater the number of people who walk through a crime scene, the greater the amount of altered or lost evidence. One of the goals of scene management is to limit the number of people moving in and out of the area of the crime.

Only those EMTs and paramedics who have to enter the scene should be present inside the scene perimeter. There must be a clearly established perimeter set up by the police. Ask about it.

Once the EMT/paramedic has entered the scene, observe the surroundings. Noting the relative position of objects in the area is important. This is particularly true if the EMT or paramedic moves anything while reaching and treating a patient. If it is a case such as a homicide where no treatment is to be given, the EMS personnel must still confirm the death of the person. That means checking the "ABCs". Accomplish this with minimal scene disruption in most instances. If the "ABCs" are not done, then do not record that the person was pulseless and without respirations.·

This does not mean that every EMS responder has to enter the scene. One member entering to confirm the death of the person is enough. Remember that every person who walks through the scene alters it and destroys more evidence.

When the prehospital care provider enters the crime scene, he must note any item touched or moved by him. Inform the officer in charge about items moved or touched. Also, enter and exit by the same pathway. Do not wander around the scene. Get the information you need, then leave. If the patient is still viable, work the patient. Nevertheless, if you move, alter or damage items by your efforts, make note of it.

At crime scenes it is usually alteration of insignificant-appearing items and circumstances which makes a difference to the investigation. For instance, opening a window can cause items to blow around in the room, altering their position. It also lets outside elements in, which can destroy evidence. Unbuttoning the shirt or loosening the collar/tie on a body allows you better access the neck. It looks trivial to you, but could throw an entire investigation off if no one tells the investigating officer.

If something that you note about the scene looks out of the ordinary, tell the police. Let them decide if it is significant. However, do not try to be a detective. Leave that to the police. They won't try to be EMTs or paramedics. They will leave that to you.

If the EMS personnel should arrive at a call and suspect that it is a crime scene, they should immediately inform the police. The EMT/paramedic has a responsibility to keep the scene secure until the arrival of the police. This could take the form of keeping unauthorized persons out of the area. The EMS personnel also should note such items as smoke and odors that are present when they arrive. The loss of such evidence may be unavoidable. Report the existence of such evidence to the police when they arrive.[74]

Do Not Resuscitate (DNR) Orders

Provision of care in the home for an increasing number of patients during their final days is becoming more common. Many times these patients present to the EMT/paramedic in cardiac arrest. The family states that resuscitation of the patient is not to be done. This presents the EMT or paramedic with a dilemma. Should the effort to resuscitate proceed, or should efforts cease? The answer is not always clear. Trying to apply a simple axiom such as "when in doubt, resuscitate" to these situations invites outright hostility from some family members. They strongly believe that their loved one wishes to die in peace. Try doing CPR. They may go so far as to physically assault you.

There is a lot to be said for death with dignity.

Who speaks for the patient? The patient cannot express his wishes at that moment. What do you do if the people on scene hand you an order not to resuscitate the patient? Is the order valid? Is it written? You have to decide immediately. You also will have to document it.

Some situations resolve easily. A member of a hospice program is in attendance. Also, another healthcare worker, such as a visiting nurse, may have the patient's record readily available. If none of these resources are present, then the EMT/paramedic may wish to proceed as outlined below.

Situations such as this might occur with more frequency as time passes. This is because the elderly population of the United States is a rapidly increasing group. There are more people and they are living longer. Many of them wish to die when their time comes. They do not wish any extraordinary measures to be taken to prolong their life. This is particularly true if they are suffering from a disease process the recovery from which exceeds the capability of current therapy.[75]

So who speaks for the patient? If the patient can speak for himself, then that is fine. What is done if the patient is unable to speak? Then the family members in communication with the physician can speak for the patient.

If it is the patient who is speaking, the patient must be competent to decide. Satisfy this test of competency by assuring the patient's understanding of the implications of the proposed action or inaction.[76] If it is the family and the physician, then the past statements made by the patient will have a bearing on the decision.[77]

Judge the validity of the written order. Consider the amount of time that has passed since the writing of the order. Determine that the patient has an illness that is irreversible and irreparable with death imminent.[78] In this patient, the chances of death occurring within two weeks are very great.[79]

It is reasonable to question the age of a DNR order, particularly one a few months old. The EMT/paramedic may have an intuitive sense that the order represents a valid wish on the part of the patient. Nevertheless, confirm the order. This may take the form of conversation with the patient's

Know what the policy of your EMS system is before being confronted with a DNR in the field.

physician. It could be with the EMS system's medical control physician. Document the situation. Remember that future inquiry into the case is possible. Some states are enacting programs using items such as bracelets similar to the Medicalert identifiers. These are easily identifiable and verifiable in the cases of DNR. Programs such as this have potential to make decision-making easier in instances where the patient is not able to speak his wishes.

Before you respond to a call, know what the expectations of the medical community are concerning your behavior. It is much better to know what you are going to do when confronted with a DNR order—much better than waiting and then having to scramble and stammer when one is suddenly thrust into your hands.

Scrutinize the axiom "when in doubt, resuscitate" more closely. It may hold true in some cases, but clearly not in all.

If, after all of this, there is still a reasonable doubt about the validity of the DNR order, then resuscitate. Make the resuscitation effort within the guidelines of the local protocols.[80]

Documenting Sudden Death

There will be times when the EMT/paramedic needs to document a sudden death. The situation could arise as a result of a response to a cardiac arrest call. The EMS personnel find a patient who is obviously dead. This is a person who is beyond the point where current therapy can intervene to return the person to a functional existence.

Prehospital personnel also encounter such instances on responses to reports of sudden death where the person died several hours or days ago (or longer). It could also be to crime scenes, such as homicide. They find that the expired person has been there for a length of time. Or else under circumstances that prohibit effective resuscitation.

The same may be true for industrial and motor vehicle accidents.

EMS, for all its potential to do good, will not conquer death. People are still going to die, and EMS will be there on occasion to witness and document it. The document created at the time by the EMT/paramedic will serve to ensure that anything reasonable was done. It also might confirm that it was unreasonable to do anything. It must stand up to future inquiry.

The future inquiry may be through the legal system and the courts. It could be through a police investigation or the medical community (including the medical examiner). Whatever its source, the answer to the inquiry must show that EMS personnel competently and professionally execute their duties. There should not be any reasonable doubt about the actions of the EMT or paramedic. Proper documentation will help to ensure this.

When faced with the task of documenting a sudden death, make two broad subdivisions. First, there are those who receive an evaluation of the situation, and no effort to resuscitate is begun. The second group are those who have an effort begun and later terminated before transporting the patient to the hospital.

In the first instance the EMT/paramedic should proceed as outlined in the section of crime scene management. Move nothing that you do not have to move. Note any movement of objects. This is particularly important at the crime scene. It is also important where the cause of death is a natural part of the person's life cycle. Respect the deceased person and his personal effects.

Protocols may vary from system to system. If the EMS system sends response units to a scene of a sudden death, there is a responsibility to document the event. Questions about the scene need answers. Questions such as who declared the person dead? How was it determined? At what time? Was there anything unusual about the circumstances? For instance, was any trauma noted? Did the person have a long-standing medical history? Who was the patient's physician? What medication did the patient regularly take?

The answers to the above questions may mean the difference between an investigation into cause of death vs. the release to a funeral director after completion of some paperwork. The effect of all this on surviving family members could be no small matter. Did their loved one die of natural causes, or was there a suspicion of foul play? It is not that the EMS personnel are acting as detectives. Nevertheless, they are observers who are present at the scene of the death. They have information to obtain and refer to authorities such as the medical examiner and law enforcement personnel.

The second group are those who have an effort to resuscitate started which is later stopped in the field. These patients are usually the recipient of advanced life support from paramedics. They may be presenting in asystole or electromechanical dissociation that does not respond to available therapies. These patients have a poor prognosis with a dismal survival rate.[81]

More EMS systems are recognizing that futile resuscitation efforts put their EMTs and paramedics at greater risk. They also drive up the cost of healthcare, and can jeopardize the public safety.

Prehospital personnel still must document the course of treatment. In all probability the EMT/paramedic still must contact the medical examiner. He also must send a report in writing to the medical examiner. A medical-legal document will exist. The document should state how the patient presented to the EMS personnel. If you make a positive identification of the patient on scene, then include the deceased's name, address, age and date of birth.

For either group, record any know history of present illness. An unwitnessed cardiac arrest is the situation for many of these responses. Sometimes non-family members make the discovery. They may know very little about the person or what happened. They will probably not know much about the past medical history either. In cases such as this, any available medication containers may shed some light on the patients history. Obviously, take note of any physical findings. Look for evidence of trauma, gastrointestinal bleeding, or vomiting. Examine for medic alert bracelets and chains.

Remember that your documentation may surface later. It could be part of an investigation. Its use also might be in litigation over such items as insurance benefits for the deceased. EMTs and paramedics are responsible for providing clear documentation of the event.

Finally, be sensitive to the emotions and needs of the survivors, be they family members, or friends or acquaintances of the deceased. Any of these people could become a patient. Also, they have emotional needs that might be met in part by caring EMS personnel responding to the call.

10

Final Remarks

This training manual presents documentation skills for the emergency medical service. Recording emergency care is a key function of the emergency medical service. Clear concise reports are the record of the findings and patient management in the field. The reports affect the care provided in the hospital. Remember that run reports provide data for research. The report reflects on the quality of the care. It is a legal record.

Report writing is a skill. Skills require practice. Skills need attention to detail. Be aware of how you report the patient care event. Form good report writing habits. Improve your reporting habits and you present yourself and the patient better.

The emergency medical service is entering its adult stage of growth. The records we leave will measure the maturity we have gained.

Section 2

Sample Run Reports & Classroom Exercises

11

Run Report Forms

The next section contains written reports. They are from a fictitious community.

There are only two hospitals in this community:

1. Trauma General Hospital is a Level 1 Trauma Center. It is capable of handling any patient brought to it. In order to do this, the hospital maintains a large staff. It always has medical and surgical specialty teams available in-house. It might be referred to as *Trauma General* or *T.G.H.* or *Trauma Gen. Hosp.* as well as *Trauma General Hospital* in the reports.

2. Community Hospital is a smaller facility with one physician staffing the Emergency Department. The Department has a staff capable of handling most of the everyday emergencies that make up 80% to 90% of all emergency cases. It might be referred to as *Community* or *C.H.* or *Comm. Hosp.* in the report forms.

Transport priorities are:

1. Immediate life-threatening

2. Urgent/Potential life threatening

3. Emergent non-life-threatening

4. Routine non-emergent transfer

The reports contain some standard items. These are:

1. BLS ambulances have the letter A as the prefix. They are staffed by EMT personnel without advanced training or skills. Their care is non-invasive. They do have automatic external defibrillators.

2. ALS ambulance have the letter P as the prefix. They are staffed by paramedics with a full range of advanced life support skills.

3. Medical Control physicians have a two-digit number.

4. Paramedics have a three-digit number ($1xx$).

5. EMTs have a three-digit number ($3xx$).

The following trip sheets are based on actual cases and the case documentation. They are from calls responded to by EMTs and paramedics in Massachusetts. Information that could identify either the patient or the author of the report has been altered to protect the privacy of the individuals.

The purpose is to expose the student to a variety of writing formats, some of which deviate greatly from the SEMS format suggested by this book. By reviewing and editing the writing samples, the reader will develop his writing skills.

The reports themselves contain diverse examples of report writing. The perfect report might not exist, but the goal is to have EMS personnel consistently writing the best report they can. With practice, your writing should improve.

Some of the reports contain grammatical and spelling errors. This is by design. Correct spelling and grammar is important. If it is worth writing about, then write about it correctly. Also, the reader will note non-standard abbreviations. At times, you will have to pause to figure out what the writer was getting at. As you do this, think of the effect the use of non-standard abbreviations in your reports have on the hospital personnel who read them. Although an abbreviation means something to you, it could look like nothing more than a jumble of letters to anyone else.

As classroom exercises, use the reports for group discussion. Take some of them and rewrite them using the principles contained in this text. You can improve on any writing. For instance, is the information complete? How well is it organized? Can you find information easily? Are some terms overused? Examples of this would be "pt. states" or "pt. denies" used repeatedly instead of combining all such statements under one heading. Is it clear to you, the reader, what went on at the call? Is it easy to find out what is wrong with the patient? Or is the chief complaint buried somewhere in the report?

Is the form filled in as completely as possible? Ask yourself what it would be like if it was your report and you had to rely on it to testify at a hearing. Ask yourself what it would be like if you had to read the report in court. Would it represent you and your services as a professional healthcare organization, or would it be an embarrassment?

The first group of reports are BLS in nature. This should not imply that ALS personnel can skip this section. All good ALS is good BLS first. This includes the ability to write a report. Some of the situations that present as BLS cases can be as challenging as those that are ALS. For example, documenting the care given to the uncooperative patient needs to be done carefully whether the provider is an EMT or a paramedic.

Some systems employ a two-tiered response. Others use only EMTs or paramedics. Regardless of system configuration, all EMS personnel do non-ALS calls. Skillful documentation is essential on all responses.

E.M.S. TRAINING PROGRAM
PATIENT CARE REPORT FORM

© 1992 Kennedy Associates

Patient Name:	Trip #: *001* Date:
Address:	M.R.#: Day:
	Dispatch To: For:
DOB: Tel. #:	
Next of Kin:	Dispatch Time: *4:00* Arrival Time: *PM*
Address:	To Hospital: At Hospital:
	Location at Dispatch:
Relationship: Tel. #:	Billing Information (circle):
Transported to: Transport Priority:	Medicare Medicaid BC/BS
Miles from: To:	Indust. Acc. Self Other
❏ No Transport	Subscriber:
REASON:	
	Policy #:

Physical Exam

Eye Opening	☒ Spontaneous ❏ To Pain	
	❏ To Voice ❏ None	
Verbal Response	❏ Oriented ❏ Confused	
	❏ Inappropriate ❏ Incomprehensible ❏ None	
Motor Response	❏ Obedience ❏ Purposeful ❏ Withdrawal	
	❏ Flexion ❏ Extension ❏ None	
Skin Condition	❏ Normal ☒ Cool ❏ Hot ❏ Pale	
	❏ Flushed ❏ Cyanotic ❏ Diaphoretic	

Chief Complaint/History/Changes in Patient Status

23 y/o male

Shot in stomach ⓁHumerus ⓁWrist

PT found in chair with bullet wounds to stomach Ⓛhumerus ⓁWrist

PT placed in shock position and given 4 Lpm O2

Vital Signs

❏ Unable to Obtain   ❏ Not attempted
REASON:

Time	BP	Pulse	Resp. Rate/Effort
		80	18 Reg

Allergies:	❏ None ❏ Unknown
Current Medications:	❏ None ☒ Unknown

Brought with Pt.? ❏ Yes ❏ No

Advanced Life Support

Time /	Medication /	Rate/Dose /	Route
/	/	/	
/	/	/	
/	/	/	
/	/	/	
/	/	/	
/	/	/	
/	/	/	

Suspected Diagnosis: ❏ Chronic ☒ Acute
☒ Major Trauma ☒ Acute Medical ❏ Cardiac Arrest ❏ Shock
❏ Minor Trauma ❏ Minor Medical ❏ Cardiac Disorder ❏ ETOH
❏ Soft Tissue Injury ❏ Burns ❏ Ortho ❏ OD/Poison
❏ Neuro ❏ Seizure ❏ Psych ❏ OB/GYN ❏ Neonate

Total Fluid Infused: mls

Emergency Care: ❏ CPR ❏ Extricate ❏ Back/Neck Immobilize
☒ Bleed Control ❏ Bandage ❏ Splint ❏ Heat/Cold Applied
❏ O₂ Administration: _____ liters/minute via _____
Airway: ❏ Cleared ❏ Oral ❏ Nasal Size: _____ ❏ Suction
Intubate: ❏ Endotracheal ❏ Nasotracheal Size: _____
Assist Ventilation: Rate: _____ Method: _____
❏ ECG Monitor ❏ Rhythm Strip Attached
Transport Position: *Shock Position*

DEFIB: Time: Time: Time: Time:	
Joules: Joules: Joules: Joules:	

Medical Control: ❏ Direct ❏ C-MED Channel _____
MD#_____ Hospital _____
Hospital Notified Enroute: ❏ Yes ❏ No
❏ C-MED ❏ Dispatcher

Other Response Units/Agencies:

Unit #	EMT/Paramedic Signatures:
	_____ # _____ _____ # _____ _____ # _____

The Write Way to Better EMS

E.M.S. TRAINING PROGRAM
PATIENT CARE REPORT FORM

© 1992 Kennedy Associat

Patient Name: **James Miller**

Address: **150 Tremont Ave**
Boston MA

DOB: **July 4 1911**   Tel. #: **555-1212**

Next of Kin: **Mary Miller**

Address: **Same**

Relationship: **Wife**   Tel. #: **Same**

Transported to: Transport Priority:

Miles from: To:

❑ No Transport
REASON:

Trip #: **002**   Date: **9-30-92**

M.R.#:   Day:

Dispatch To: **150 Tremont Ave** For: **Injury**

Dispatch Time: Arrival Time:

To Hospital: At Hospital:

Location at Dispatch:

Billing Information (circle): **(Medicare)**   Medicaid   BC/BS
Indust. Acc.   Self   Other

Subscriber: **James Miller**
S/A

Policy #:

Physical Exam

Eye Opening	❑ Spontaneous ❑ To Pain	❑ To Voice ❑ None
Verbal Response	❑ Oriented ❑ Confused	❑ Inappropriate ❑ Incomprehensible ❑ None
Motor Response	❑ Obedience ❑ Purposeful ❑ Withdrawal	❑ Flexion ❑ Extension ❑ None
Skin Condition	❑ Normal ❑ Cool ❑ Hot ❑ Pale	❑ Flushed ❑ Cyanotic ❑ Diaphoretic

Vital Signs

❑ Unable to Obtain   ❑ Not attempted
REASON:

Time	BP	Pulse	Resp. Rate/Effort

Allergies: ❑ None   ❑ Unknown

Current Medications: ❑ None   ❑ Unknown

Brought with Pt.?   ❑ Yes   ❑ No

Suspected Diagnosis: ❑ Chronic   ❑ Acute
❑ Major Trauma ❑ Acute Medical ❑ Cardiac Arrest ❑ Shock
❑ Minor Trauma ❑ Minor Medical ❑ Cardiac Disorder ❑ ETOH
❑ Soft Tissue Injury ❑ Burns ❑ Ortho ❑ OD/Poison
❑ Neuro ❑ Seizure ❑ Psych ❑ OB/GYN ❑ Neonate

Emergency Care: ❑ CPR ❑ Extricate ☒ Back/Neck Immobilize
❑ Bleed Control ❑ Bandage ❑ Splint ❑ Heat/Cold Applied
❑ O₂ Administration: _____ liters/minute via _____
Airway: ❑ Cleared ❑ Oral ❑ Nasal Size: _____ ❑ Suction
Intubate: ❑ Endotracheal ❑ Nasotracheal Size: _____
Assist Ventilation: Rate: _____ Method: _____
❑ ECG Monitor ❑ Rhythm Strip Attached
Transport Position: **Stretcher**

Chief Complaint/History/Changes in Patient Status

81 year old ♂
Pt Fell down stairs
c/o pain → neck   C≠A

Advanced Life Support

Time	/	Medication	/	Rate/Dose	/	Route
/			/		/	
/			/		/	
/			/		/	
/			/		/	
/			/		/	
/			/		/	
/			/		/	

Total Fluid Infused: _____ mls

DEFIB: Time: Time: Time: Time:
Joules: Joules: Joules: Joules:

Medical Control: ❑ Direct ❑ C-MED Channel _____
MD#_____   Hospital _____
Hospital Notified Enroute: ❑ Yes   ❑ No
❑ C-MED ❑ Dispatcher

Other Response Units/Agencies:

Unit # **A20**   EMT/Paramedic Signatures:
#_____   #_____   #_____

E.M.S. TRAINING PROGRAM
PATIENT CARE REPORT FORM

© 1992 Kennedy Associates

Patient Name: Camille Dill	Trip #: 003 Date: Sept. 30 1992
Address: 7 Olive Ave	M.R.#: Day: Wednesday
Readville MA	Dispatch To: 7 Olive Ave For:
DOB: Sept. 30, 1968 Tel. #:	1st floor
Next of Kin:	Dispatch Time: Arrival Time:
Address:	To Hospital: At Hospital:
	Location at Dispatch:

Relationship: Tel. #:

Billing Information (circle):
Medicare   Medicaid   BC/BS
Indust. Acc.   Self   Other

Transported to: Transport Priority:

Miles from: To:

☒ No Transport
REASON: Patient Refusal

Subscriber:

Policy #:

Physical Exam

Eye Opening	☒ Spontaneous ☐ To Pain	
	☐ To Voice ☐ None	
Verbal Response	☐ Oriented ☐ Confused	
	☐ Inappropriate ☐ Incomprehensible ☐ None	
Motor Response	☐ Obedience ☐ Purposeful ☐ Withdrawal	
	☐ Flexion ☐ Extension ☐ None	
Skin Condition	☐ Normal ☐ Cool ☐ Hot ☐ Pale	
	☐ Flushed ☐ Cyanotic ☐ Diaphoretic	

Vital Signs

☒ Unable to Obtain   ☐ Not attempted
REASON: uncooperative

Time	BP	Pulse	Resp. Rate/Effort
		60-70	16 regular

Allergies: ☐ None ☐ Unknown

Current Medications: ☐ None ☐ Unknown

Brought with Pt.?   ☐ Yes   ☐ No

Suspected Diagnosis: ☐ Chronic   ☐ Acute
☐ Major Trauma ☐ Acute Medical ☐ Cardiac Arrest ☐ Shock
☐ Minor Trauma ☐ Minor Medical ☐ Cardiac Disorder ☐ ETOH
☐ Soft Tissue Injury ☐ Burns ☐ Ortho ☐ OD/Poison
☐ Neuro ☐ Seizure ☐ Psych ☐ OB/GYN ☐ Neonate

Chief Complaint/History/Changes in Patient Status

24 year old female found standing on her own upon arrival turned and walked to rocking chair sat down and in my opinion faked unconsciousness. Pt responds immedrately to ammonia and refused transport x3 (family was agitated from the moment we arrived)

Advanced Life Support

Time /	Medication /	Rate/Dose /	Route
/	/	/	
/	/	/	
/	/	/	
/	/	/	
/	/	/	
/	/	/	
/	/	/	
/	/	/	

Total Fluid Infused: mls

Emergency Care: ☐ CPR ☐ Extricate ☐ Back/Neck Immobilize
☐ Bleed Control ☐ Bandage ☐ Splint ☐ Heat/Cold Applied
☐ O₂ Administration: _____ liters/minute via _____
Airway: ☐ Cleared ☐ Oral ☐ Nasal Size: _____ ☐ Suction
Intubate: ☐ Endotracheal ☐ Nasotracheal Size: _____
Assist Ventilation: Rate: _____ Method: _____
☐ ECG Monitor ☐ Rhythm Strip Attached
Transport Position:

DEFIB: Time:	Time:	Time:	Time:
Joules:	Joules:	Joules:	Joules:

Medical Control: ☐ Direct ☐ C-MED Channel _____
MD#_____ Hospital _____
Hospital Notified Enroute: ☐ Yes ☐ No
☐ C-MED ☐ Dispatcher

Other Response Units/Agencies:

Unit # A35

EMT/Paramedic Signatures:
John Task # 305   Ed T. # 310   #

E.M.S. TRAINING PROGRAM
PATIENT CARE REPORT FORM

© 1992 Kennedy Associate

Patient Name: Mary Peterson	Trip #: 004 Date: 9-30-92
Address: 15 Apple Hill Lane	M.R.#: Day: Wed
Nahant, MA	Dispatch To: For: unconsious
DOB: 6-18-70 Tel. #: 555-8828	Main St. Station
Next of Kin: John Keller	Dispatch Time: 1701 Arrival Time:
Address: Same	To Hospital: At Hospital:
	Location at Dispatch:
Relationship: Boyfriend Tel. #:	Billing Information (circle):
Transported to: Community Hosp. Transport Priority:	
Miles from: 906.4 To: 2	Medicare Medicaid BC/BS
❏ No Transport	Indust. Acc. (Self) Other
REASON:	Subscriber:
	Policy #:

Physical Exam

Eye Opening	☒ Spontaneous ❏ To Pain
	❏ To Voice ❏ None
Verbal Response	☒ Oriented ❏ Confused
	❏ Inappropriate ❏ Incomprehensible ❏ None
Motor Response	☒ Obedience ❏ Purposeful ❏ Withdrawal
	❏ Flexion ❏ Extension ❏ None
Skin Condition	☒ Normal ❏ Cool ❏ Hot ❏ Pale
	❏ Flushed ❏ Cyanotic ❏ Diaphoretic

Vital Signs

❏ Unable to Obtain   ❏ Not attempted

REASON:

Time	BP	Pulse	Resp. Rate/Effort
1714	116/74	88 R	16 c/r

Allergies: ❏ None
    Dilantin   ❏ Unknown
Current Medications: ❏ None
    Tegretol, Klonapin, Prozac   ❏ Unknown

Brought with Pt.? ❏ Yes ❏ No

Suspected Diagnosis: ❏ Chronic   ❏ Acute
❏ Major Trauma ❏ Acute Medical ❏ Cardiac Arrest ❏ Shock
❏ Minor Trauma ❏ Minor Medical ❏ Cardiac Disorder ❏ ETOH
❏ Soft Tissue Injury ❏ Burns ❏ Ortho ❏ OD/Poison
❏ Neuro ❏ Seizure ❏ Psych ❏ OB/GYN ❏ Neonate

Chief Complaint/History/Changes in Patient Status

22 y/o ♀ supine on floor at subway station after witnessed (petit mal) seizure approx 1-2 min long. Pt. + boyfriend both state she has seizures all the time but today 8 seizures. Pt just seen and discharged from Hosp. + on her way home.

PE: CA+Ox3, skin warm+dry pup =+react @ 3mm Head + Neck ⊖ Chest sym c̄ =bilat lung sounds ABD + Pelvis ⊖ ROM x 4.

PMH: C.P., seizures + depression
MEDS: as listed   NKDA
    Pt suffered 3 petit mall Sx during trans to Hospital
Pt CA+Ox3 immed after each

Advanced Life Support

Time /	Medication /	Rate/Dose /	Route
/	/	/	
/	/	/	
/	/	/	
/	/	/	
/	/	/	
/	/	/	
/	/	/	
/	/	/	

Total Fluid Infused: mls

Emergency Care: ❏ CPR ❏ Extricate ❏ Back/Neck Immobilize
❏ Bleed Control ❏ Bandage ❏ Splint ❏ Heat/Cold Applied
❏ O₂ Administration: _____ liters/minute via _____
Airway: ❏ Cleared ❏ Oral ❏ Nasal Size: _____ ❏ Suction
Intubate: ❏ Endotracheal ❏ Nasotracheal Size: _____
Assist Ventilation: Rate: _____ Method: _____
❏ ECG Monitor ❏ Rhythm Strip Attached
Transport Position: Semi-fowlers

DEFIB: Time:	Time:	Time:	Time:
Joules:	Joules:	Joules:	Joules:

Medical Control: ❏ Direct ❏ C-MED Channel _____
MD#_____   Hospital _____
Hospital Notified Enroute: ❏ Yes ☒ No
    ❏ C-MED ❏ Dispatcher

Other Response Units/Agencies:
    Police

Unit # A42   EMT/Paramedic Signatures:
Carl Nelson   # 325 _____   F.C. # 350 _____   # _____

E.M.S. TRAINING PROGRAM
PATIENT CARE REPORT FORM

© 1992 Kennedy Associates

Patient Name: Julia Ritter	Trip #: 005 Date: 9-30-92
Address: 10 Francis St	M.R.#: 020 58 64 1 Day:
Medford MA	Dispatch To: For: Leg Pain
DOB: Feb 3, 1911 Tel. #: 555-6432	10 Francis St.
Next of Kin:	Dispatch Time: 0945 Arrival Time: 1005
Address:	To Hospital: 1015 At Hospital: 1030
	Location at Dispatch: Station 2

Relationship: Tel. #:

Billing Information (circle):

Transported to: Community Hosp   Transport Priority: 3

Miles from: To:

(Medicare)   Medicaid   BC/BS
Indust. Acc.   Self   Other

❑ No Transport
REASON:

Subscriber: Patient

Policy #:

Physical Exam

Eye Opening	❑ Spontaneous ❑ To Pain	
	❑ To Voice ❑ None	
Verbal Response	❑ Oriented ❑ Confused	
	❑ Inappropriate ❑ Incomprehensible ❑ None	
Motor Response	❑ Obedience ❑ Purposeful ❑ Withdrawal	
	❑ Flexion ❑ Extension ❑ None	
Skin Condition	☒ Normal ❑ Cool ❑ Hot ❑ Pale	
	❑ Flushed ❑ Cyanotic ❑ Diaphoretic	

Chief Complaint/History/Changes in Patient Status

81 yo ♀ s/p bilateral amputation last surgery Ⓛ leg 12/91 % severe pain both stumps Ø relief w̄ percocet Pt has hx of vascular Disease Bilaterally legs resulting in amputation of knee. Is Depressed has Pacemaker, chronic pain meds- Isordil HCTZ, clonidine, folic acid prozac ferrous sulfate Trazadone Xanat, fer

Vital Signs

❑ Unable to Obtain   ❑ Not attempted
REASON:

Time	BP	Pulse	Resp. Rate/Effort
	80/56	68	18

Allergies: NKA   ☒ None   ❑ Unknown

Current Medications: ❑ None   ❑ Unknown

See above

Brought with Pt.? ❑ Yes ❑ No

Suspected Diagnosis: ❑ Chronic ❑ Acute
❑ Major Trauma ❑ Acute Medical ❑ Cardiac Arrest ❑ Shock
❑ Minor Trauma ❑ Minor Medical ❑ Cardiac Disorder ❑ ETOH
❑ Soft Tissue Injury ❑ Burns ❑ Ortho ❑ OD/Poison
❑ Neuro ❑ Seizure ❑ Psych ❑ OB/GYN ❑ Neonate

Advanced Life Support

Time	/	Medication	/	Rate/Dose	/	Route
	/		/		/	
	/		/		/	
	/		/		/	
	/		/		/	
	/		/		/	
	/		/		/	
	/		/		/	

Total Fluid Infused: mls

Emergency Care: ❑ CPR ❑ Extricate ❑ Back/Neck Immobilize
❑ Bleed Control ❑ Bandage ❑ Splint ❑ Heat/Cold Applied
❑ O₂ Administration: _____ liters/minute via _____
Airway: ❑ Cleared ❑ Oral ❑ Nasal Size: _____ ❑ Suction
Intubate: ❑ Endotracheal ❑ Nasotracheal Size: _____
Assist Ventilation: Rate: _____ Method: _____
❑ ECG Monitor ❑ Rhythm Strip Attached
Transport Position: Full Fowlers

DEFIB: Time:	Time:	Time:	Time:
Joules:	Joules:	Joules:	Joules:

Medical Control: ❑ Direct ❑ C-MED Channel _____
MD#_____ Hospital _____
Hospital Notified Enroute: ❑ Yes ❑ No
❑ C-MED ❑ Dispatcher

Other Response Units/Agencies:

Unit #	EMT/Paramedic Signatures:
A54	Thomas Martin # 327 Frank Joy # 345 _____ #

E.M.S. TRAINING PROGRAM
PATIENT CARE REPORT FORM

© 1992 Kennedy Associate

Patient Name: Robert Smith (? of from ID)	Trip #: 006 Date: Sept 30 '92
Address: 18 Church St	M.R.#: 501 28 01 Day:
Haverhill MA	Dispatch To: For: Seizure
DOB: Tel. #: 555 7863	10th Ave + 42nd St
Next of Kin: Unknown	Dispatch Time: Arrival Time:
Address:	To Hospital: At Hospital:
	Location at Dispatch:
Relationship: Tel. #:	Billing Information (circle):
Transported to: TGH Transport Priority:	Medicare (Medicaid) BC/BS
Miles from: To:	Indust. Acc. Self Other
❏ No Transport	Subscriber:
REASON:	
	Policy #:

Physical Exam

Eye Opening	☑ Spontaneous ❏ To Pain	
	❏ To Voice ❏ None	
Verbal Response	❏ Oriented ☑ Confused	
	❏ Inappropriate ❏ Incomprehensible ❏ None	
Motor Response	☑ Obedience ❏ Purposeful ❏ Withdrawal	
	❏ Flexion ❏ Extension ❏ None	
Skin Condition	❏ Normal ❏ Cool ❏ Hot ❏ Pale	
	❏ Flushed ❏ Cyanotic ☑ Diaphoretic	

Chief Complaint/History/Changes in Patient Status

Seizure
38 yo ♂ SZ. activity for @ 4 mins.
Now confused to day/date.
∅ incontinence —
PMH: SXRS
Rx: DILANTIN. (non compliant)
All: NKA
∅ oral trauma
        Last drink yesterday
at @ noon.
Tx: Transport s̄ ∆

Vital Signs

❏ Unable to Obtain   ❏ Not attempted
REASON:

Time	BP	Pulse	Resp. Rate/Effort
@ 0519	134/62	120	16

Allergies: ❏ None
                              ❏ Unknown

Current Medications: ❏ None
                              ❏ Unknown

Brought with Pt.?   ❏ Yes   ❏ No

Suspected Diagnosis: ❏ Chronic   ❏ Acute
❏ Major Trauma ❏ Acute Medical ❏ Cardiac Arrest ❏ Shock
❏ Minor Trauma ❏ Minor Medical ❏ Cardiac Disorder ❏ ETOH
❏ Soft Tissue Injury ❏ Burns ❏ Ortho ❏ OD/Poison
❏ Neuro ☒ Seizure ❏ Psych ❏ OB/GYN ❏ Neonate

Advanced Life Support

Time	/	Medication	/	Rate/Dose	/	Route
	/		/		/	
	/		/		/	
	/		/		/	
	/		/		/	
	/		/		/	
	/		/		/	

Total Fluid Infused: mls

Emergency Care: ❏ CPR ❏ Extricate ❏ Back/Neck Immobilize
❏ Bleed Control ❏ Bandage ❏ Splint ❏ Heat/Cold Applied
❏ O₂ Administration: _____ liters/minute via _____
Airway: ❏ Cleared ❏ Oral ❏ Nasal Size: _____ ❏ Suction
Intubate: ❏ Endotracheal ❏ Nasotracheal Size: _____
Assist Ventilation: Rate: _____ Method: _____
❏ ECG Monitor ❏ Rhythm Strip Attached
Transport Position:

DEFIB:	Time:	Time:	Time:	Time:
	Joules:	Joules:	Joules:	Joules:

Medical Control: ❏ Direct ❏ C-MED Channel _____
MD#_____ Hospital _____
Hospital Notified Enroute: ❏ Yes   ❏ No
                              ❏ C-MED ❏ Dispatcher

Other Response Units/Agencies:

Unit # A62   EMT/Paramedic Signatures:
              JK   #   _____ #   _____ #

E.M.S. TRAINING PROGRAM
PATIENT CARE REPORT FORM

© 1992 Kennedy Associates

Patient Name: Joseph Talbot	Trip #: 007 Date:
Address: 215 Hawthorne Ave	M.R.#: 600 40 20 5 Day:
Lynn MA	Dispatch To: For: MVA
DOB: Tel. #: 555-5078	Main + Minot
Next of Kin: Karen Talbot	Dispatch Time: Arrival Time:
Address: 215 Hawthorne Ave	To Hospital: At Hospital:
Lynn MA	Location at Dispatch:
Relationship: Wife Tel. #: Same	Billing Information (circle):

Transported to: Community Hosp   Transport Priority:

Miles from: To:

Billing Information (circle): Medicare   Medicaid   (BC/BS)
(Indust. Acc.) ??   Self   Other

❑ No Transport
REASON:

Subscriber: City Taxi
206 N Main St
Lynn MA
Policy #:

Physical Exam

Eye Opening	☑ Spontaneous ❑ To Pain	
	❑ To Voice ❑ None	
Verbal Response	☑ Oriented ❑ Confused	
	❑ Inappropriate ❑ Incomprehensible ❑ None	
Motor Response	☑ Obedience ❑ Purposeful ❑ Withdrawal	
	❑ Flexion ❑ Extension ❑ None	
Skin Condition	☑ Normal ❑ Cool ❑ Hot ❑ Pale	
	❑ Flushed ❑ Cyanotic ❑ Diaphoretic	

Chief Complaint/History/Changes in Patient Status

① Ⓛ Side pain S/P MVA
35 y/o ♂ unseatbelted driver of taxi
in slow moving traffic that was
rear ended by another vehicle. minor
damage to taxi
Denies LOC. C/o Pain to entire
Ⓛ side of body. No visible injuries
moves all extremities well.
Remaing exam ∅
∅ pmh   ∅ Rx   NKA
TX: C-spine immobilize
Transport ∄

Vital Signs

❑ Unable to Obtain   ❑ Not attempted
REASON:

Time	BP	Pulse	Resp. Rate/Effort
	150/P	64 R	20

Allergies: ☑ None
          ❑ Unknown

Current Medications: ☑ None
          ❑ Unknown

Brought with Pt.?   ❑ Yes   ❑ No

Suspected Diagnosis: ❑ Chronic   ❑ Acute
❑ Major Trauma ❑ Acute Medical ❑ Cardiac Arrest ❑ Shock
☑ Minor Trauma ❑ Minor Medical ❑ Cardiac Disorder ❑ ETOH
❑ Soft Tissue Injury ❑ Burns ❑ Ortho ❑ OD/Poison
❑ Neuro ❑ Seizure ❑ Psych ❑ OB/GYN ❑ Neonate

Emergency Care: ❑ CPR ❑ Extricate ☑ Back/Neck Immobilize
❑ Bleed Control ❑ Bandage ❑ Splint ❑ Heat/Cold Applied
❑ O₂ Administration: _____ liters/minute via _____
Airway: ❑ Cleared ❑ Oral ❑ Nasal Size: _____ ❑ Suction
Intubate: ❑ Endotracheal ❑ Nasotracheal Size: _____
Assist Ventilation: Rate: _____ Method: _____
❑ ECG Monitor ❑ Rhythm Strip Attached
Transport Position: Supine / long board

Advanced Life Support

Time	Medication	Rate/Dose	Route
/	/	/	
/	/	/	
/	/	/	
/	/	/	
/	/	/	
/	/	/	
/	/	/	
/	/	/	

Total Fluid Infused: _____ mls

DEFIB: Time:	Time:	Time:	Time:
Joules:	Joules:	Joules:	Joules:

Medical Control: ❑ Direct ❑ C-MED Channel _____
MD#_____ Hospital _____
Hospital Notified Enroute: ❑ Yes   ❑ No
         ❑ C-MED ❑ Dispatcher

Other Response Units/Agencies:

Unit # A54   EMT/Paramedic Signatures: J. McDonald # _____   Steve Jance # _____   # _____

E.M.S. TRAINING PROGRAM
PATIENT CARE REPORT FORM

© 1992 Kennedy Associates

Patient Name: Unknown ♂ Male	Trip #: 008	Date: 30 Sept '92
Address: Unknown	M.R.#: 650 20 35 5	Day: W
	Dispatch To:	For: Cardiac arrest
DOB: Tel. #:		
Next of Kin:	Dispatch Time:	Arrival Time:
Address:	To Hospital:	At Hospital:
	Location at Dispatch:	
Relationship: Tel. #:	Billing Information (circle):	
Transported to: TGH Transport Priority: 2	Medicare Medicaid BC/BS	
Miles from: To:	Indust. Acc. Self Other	
☐ No Transport	Subscriber: No Information Available	
REASON:	Policy #:	

Physical Exam

Eye Opening	☐ Spontaneous	☐ To Pain
	☑ To Voice	☐ None
Verbal Response	☐ Oriented	☐ Confused
	☑ Inappropriate	☐ Incomprehensible ☐ None
Motor Response	☐ Obedience	☑ Purposeful ☐ Withdrawal
	☐ Flexion	☐ Extension ☐ None
Skin Condition	☑ Normal ☐ Cool ☐ Hot ☐ Pale	
	☐ Flushed ☐ Cyanotic ☐ Diaphoretic	

Vital Signs

☐ Unable to Obtain   ☐ Not attempted
REASON:

Time	BP	Pulse	Resp. Rate/Effort
0	100/70	124	24
0	130/p	120	—

Allergies: unkn   ☐ None ☐ Unknown

Current Medications: unkn   ☐ None ☐ Unknown

Brought with Pt.?   ☐ Yes   ☐ No

Suspected Diagnosis: ☐ Chronic ☑ Acute
☐ Major Trauma ☑ Acute Medical ☐ Cardiac Arrest ☐ Shock
☐ Minor Trauma ☐ Minor Medical ☐ Cardiac Disorder ☐ ETOH
☐ Soft Tissue Injury ☐ Burns ☐ Ortho ☐ OD/Poison
☑ Neuro ☐ Seizure ☐ Psych ☐ OB/GYN ☐ Neonate

Emergency Care: ☐ CPR ☐ Extricate ☐ Back/Neck Immobilize
☐ Bleed Control ☐ Bandage ☐ Splint ☐ Heat/Cold Applied
☑ O₂ Administration: 15 liters/minute via NRB
Airway: ☐ Cleared ☐ Oral ☐ Nasal Size: _____ ☐ Suction
Intubate: ☐ Endotracheal ☐ Nasotracheal Size: _____
Assist Ventilation: Rate: _____ Method: _____
☐ ECG Monitor ☐ Rhythm Strip Attached
Transport Position: LLR

Chief Complaint/History/Changes in Patient Status

82 y/o ♂ found supine on sidewalk c̄ Fire Dept on scene. Pt. unresponsive initially Pt c̄ small abrasion L posterior head: Bright red blood from R Ear: Pt was witnessed to have 1sx Lasting unkn duration: Pt then fell: Pt s̄ obvious depression or other deformity PERL Approx 4mm: Pt s̄ obvious palpable deformity to C-spine: No Pain upon Exa Trach midline No JVD noted: Pt fully C-spine immobilized for precaution Pt placed on High Flow O₂ V.S. as noted: Chest symetrical ↑↓ Abd: soft Non Ten No pulsating masses noted: Pelvis intact distal pulses intact. during Transferring Pt to Amb Pt Vommited Approx 600 cc dark vomittus: Pt rolled on L side to maintain airway suctioned another 100 from oropharynx Pt c̄ ↑ M.S. during transpo to Hosp: EMTs were told on scene

Advanced Life Support

Time /	Medication /	Rate/Dose /	Route
Pt c̄ PMH: Old Head bleed! ON			
Dilantin/Tegretol// Methyledopa			
HCTZ Diazide Motrin: Allergies NKA			
Pt transported To Hosp S A			
/	/	/	
/	/	/	
/	/	/	

Total Fluid Infused: _____ mls

DEFIB: Time:	Time:	Time:	Time:
Joules:	Joules:	Joules:	Joules:

Medical Control: ☐ Direct ☐ C-MED Channel 7
MD#_____ Hospital _____
Hospital Notified Enroute: ☑ Yes ☐ No
   ☑ C-MED ☐ Dispatcher

Other Response Units/Agencies:
Police / Fire

Unit #: A 18	EMT/Paramedic Signatures:
	Lawrence Mathew # 395 Kris Fox # 395 _____ #

E.M.S. TRAINING PROGRAM
PATIENT CARE REPORT FORM

© 1992 Kennedy Associates

Patient Name: michael Farnham	Trip #: 009 Date: 9/92
Address: 61 Webster Ave	M.R.#: Day:
Brockton mA	Dispatch To: For: Injury
DOB: Tel. #: 555-9864	61 Webster Ave Basement
Next of Kin:	Dispatch Time: Arrival Time:
Address:	To Hospital: At Hospital:
	Location at Dispatch:
Relationship: Tel. #:	Billing Information (circle):
Transported to: C.H. Transport Priority: 3	Medicare Medicaid BC/BS
Miles from: 6004.5 To: 6011.2	Indust. Acc. (Self) Other
❑ No Transport	Subscriber: Patient
REASON:	Policy #:

Physical Exam

Eye Opening	☑ Spontaneous	❑ To Pain
	❑ To Voice	❑ None
Verbal Response	☑ Oriented	❑ Confused
	❑ Inappropriate	❑ Incomprehensible ❑ None
Motor Response	☑ Obedience	❑ Purposeful ❑ Withdrawal
	❑ Flexion	❑ Extension ❑ None
Skin Condition	☑ Normal ❑ Cool ❑ Hot ❑ Pale	
	❑ Flushed ❑ Cyanotic ❑ Diaphoretic	

Chief Complaint/History/Changes in Patient Status

38 y o o ♂ found seated @ abv. who while attempting to move "keg of Beer" twisted & strained Lumbar reg. w/intermittent episodes of Pain radiating ↓ ⓛ leg. Minor muscle spasms ⓛ lateral lumbar reg. Further unrem.
PMH: ∅
Med: ∅
Aller: ∅

Vital Signs

❑ Unable to Obtain   ❑ Not attempted
REASON:

Time	BP	Pulse	Resp. Rate/Effort
1619	142/82	76	18

Allergies: ☑ None ❑ Unknown

Current Medications: ☑ None ❑ Unknown

Brought with Pt.?   ❑ Yes   ❑ No

Suspected Diagnosis: ❑ Chronic   ❑ Acute
❑ Major Trauma ❑ Acute Medical ❑ Cardiac Arrest ❑ Shock
❑ Minor Trauma ❑ Minor Medical ❑ Cardiac Disorder ❑ ETOH
☑ Soft Tissue Injury ❑ Burns ☑ Ortho ❑ OD/Poison
❑ Neuro ❑ Seizure ❑ Psych ❑ OB/GYN ❑ Neonate

Advanced Life Support

Time	/	Medication	/	Rate/Dose	/	Route
	/		/		/	
	/		/		/	
	/		/		/	
	/		/		/	
	/		/		/	
	/		/		/	
	/		/		/	

Total Fluid Infused: mls

Emergency Care: ❑ CPR ❑ Extricate ❑ Back/Neck Immobilize
❑ Bleed Control ❑ Bandage ❑ Splint ❑ Heat/Cold Applied
❑ O₂ Administration: _____ liters/minute via _____
Airway: ❑ Cleared ❑ Oral ❑ Nasal Size: _____ ❑ Suction
Intubate: ❑ Endotracheal ❑ Nasotracheal Size: _____
Assist Ventilation: Rate: _____ Method: _____
❑ ECG Monitor ❑ Rhythm Strip Attached
Transport Position:

DEFIB: Time:	Time:	Time:	Time:
Joules:	Joules:	Joules:	Joules:

Medical Control: ❑ Direct ❑ C-MED Channel _____
MD# _____ Hospital _____
Hospital Notified Enroute: ❑ Yes   ❑ No
❑ C-MED ❑ Dispatcher
Other Response Units/Agencies:

Unit # A25   EMT/Paramedic Signatures: Smith # _____   Francis # _____   # _____

E.M.S. TRAINING PROGRAM
PATIENT CARE REPORT FORM

© 1992 Kennedy Associate

Patient Name: Elizabeth Dresser	Trip #: 010 Date: 09·30·92
Address: 31 Wade Ter.	M.R.#: Day:
Cambridge MA	Dispatch To: For: Respiratory
DOB: 04-16-17 Tel. #: 555-0353	31 Wade Ter 3rd floor
Next of Kin:	Dispatch Time: Arrival Time:
Address:	To Hospital: At Hospital:
	Location at Dispatch:
Relationship: Tel. #:	Billing Information (Circle):
Transported to: C·H· Transport Priority: 2	(Medicare) Medicaid BC/BS
Miles from: To:	Indust. Acc. Self Other
❏ No Transport	Subscriber:
REASON:	
	Policy #:

Physical Exam

Eye Opening	☒ Spontaneous ❏ To Pain
	❏ To Voice ❏ None
Verbal Response	☒ Oriented ❏ Confused
	❏ Inappropriate ❏ Incomprehensible ❏ None
Motor Response	☒ Obedience ❏ Purposeful ❏ Withdrawal
	❏ Flexion ❏ Extension ❏ None
Skin Condition	❏ Normal ❏ Cool ❏ Hot ☒ Pale
	❏ Flushed ❏ Cyanotic ❏ Diaphoretic

Chief Complaint/History/Changes in Patient Status

PT is 75 y.o. ♀ C+A+0x3 PT presenting
SOB ∅ CP. R=36-40 BP 190/76 P=88
PT placed on 15l NRB in full fowlers
position. In Route, PT had less diff.
breathing R=32 BP 180/P P=80
PT tx'd → Hosp c̄ ∅ Tr̄s incident
past history CHF 30% of lung
CVA Seizures

Vital Signs

❏ Unable to Obtain   ❏ Not attempted
REASON:

Time	BP	Pulse	Resp. Rate/Effort
	190/76	88	36

Allergies: PCN	❏ None ❏ Unknown
Current Medications: Proventil	❏ None ❏ Unknown
Dilantin Digoxin	
Flourrsimide Coumadin	
Brought with Pt.? ❏ Yes ❏ No	

Advanced Life Support

Time	/	Medication	/	Rate/Dose	/	Route
	/		/		/	
	/		/		/	
	/		/		/	
	/		/		/	
	/		/		/	
	/		/		/	
	/		/		/	
	/		/		/	

Suspected Diagnosis: ❏ Chronic ❏ Acute
❏ Major Trauma ❏ Acute Medical ❏ Cardiac Arrest ❏ Shock
❏ Minor Trauma ❏ Minor Medical ❏ Cardiac Disorder ❏ ETOH
❏ Soft Tissue Injury ❏ Burns ❏ Ortho ❏ OD/Poison
❏ Neuro ❏ Seizure ❏ Psych ❏ OB/GYN ❏ Neonate

Total Fluid Infused: mls

Emergency Care: ❏ CPR ❏ Extricate ❏ Back/Neck Immobilize
❏ Bleed Control ❏ Bandage ❏ Splint ❏ Heat/Cold Applied
☒ O₂ Administration: 15 liters/minute via NRB
Airway: ❏ Cleared ❏ Oral ❏ Nasal Size: _____ ❏ Suction
Intubate: ❏ Endotracheal ❏ Nasotracheal Size: _____
Assist Ventilation: Rate: _____ Method: _____
❏ ECG Monitor ❏ Rhythm Strip Attached
Transport Position: full fowlers

DEFIB: Time:	Time:	Time:	Time:
Joules:	Joules:	Joules:	Joules:

Medical Control: ❏ Direct ❏ C-MED Channel _____
MD# _____   Hospital _____
Hospital Notified Enroute: ❏ Yes ❏ No
❏ C-MED ❏ Dispatcher

Other Response Units/Agencies:

Unit # A44 EMT/Paramedic Signatures: Cyril Ericson # 352   J.B. # 358   #

E.M.S. TRAINING PROGRAM
PATIENT CARE REPORT FORM

© 1992 Kennedy Associates

Patient Name: Richard Cabral

Address: 480 Shawmut St
Boston MA

DOB: 2-2-62   Tel. #: 555-0207

Next of Kin: Josephine Cabral

Address: Same

Relationship: Mother   Tel. #:

Transported to: Community   Transport Priority: 3

Miles from: 805.3   To: 808.4

❏ No Transport

REASON:

Trip #: 011   Date: 9-30-92

M.R.#: 060 50 30 1   Day: Wednesday

Dispatch To: For: Injury

Columbus Rd/Sunset St.

Dispatch Time: 2254   Arrival Time: 2257

To Hospital: 2310   At Hospital: 2315

Location at Dispatch: Fort Sq.

Billing Information (circle):
Medicare   Medicaid   BC/BS
Indust. Acc.   (Self)   Other

Subscriber:

Policy #:

Physical Exam

Eye Opening: ☑ Spontaneous ❏ To Pain ❏ To Voice ❏ None

Verbal Response: ☑ Oriented ❏ Confused ❏ Inappropriate ❏ Incomprehensible ❏ None

Motor Response: ☑ Obedience ❏ Purposeful ❏ Withdrawal ❏ Flexion ❏ Extension ❏ None

Skin Condition: ☑ Normal ❏ Cool ❏ Hot ❏ Pale ❏ Flushed ❏ Cyanotic ❏ Diaphoretic

Vital Signs

❏ Unable to Obtain   ❏ Not attempted

REASON:

Time	BP	Pulse	Resp. Rate/Effort
2300	138/88	116	16 c/c

Allergies: NKDA   ☑ None ❏ Unknown

Current Medications: denies   ☑ None ❏ Unknown

Brought with Pt.? ❏ Yes ❏ No

Suspected Diagnosis: ❏ Chronic ❏ Acute
❏ Major Trauma ❏ Acute Medical ❏ Cardiac Arrest ❏ Shock
❏ Minor Trauma ❏ Minor Medical ❏ Cardiac Disorder ☑ ETOH
☑ Soft Tissue Injury ❏ Burns ❏ Ortho ❏ OD/Poison
❏ Neuro ❏ Seizure ❏ Psych ❏ OB/GYN ❏ Neonate

Emergency Care: ❏ CPR ❏ Extricate ☑ Back/Neck Immobilize
❏ Bleed Control ☑ Bandage ❏ Splint ❏ Heat/Cold Applied
❏ O₂ Administration: _____ liters/minute via _____
Airway: ❏ Cleared ❏ Oral ❏ Nasal Size: _____ ❏ Suction
Intubate: ❏ Endotracheal ❏ Nasotracheal Size: _____
Assist Ventilation: Rate: _____ Method: _____
❏ ECG Monitor ❏ Rhythm Strip Attached
Transport Position: Boarded

Chief Complaint/History/Changes in Patient Status

30 yo ♂ found c̄ Fire Dept. on scene sitting on street after being struck on the head c̄ a heavy brass lamp (table type). Pt had poor recall of events prior to t after assault. ? L.O.C. Pt denies Head, neck or back pain Pt admits 16 pints of beer tonight. Ø complaint stating in slurred speech "I'm ok" uncooperative PE: C+A but slurred speech + verbally aggressive. Skin warm and dry Pupils ® reg. @ 4mm - Ⓛ slow @ 4mm. Head showed 4" LAC ® occipital reg. neck ⊖ for lacs, hemat. or PN on palp. Chest sym. c̄ = Bilateral lung sounds. abd + pelvis ⊖. Rom x y ? PMH ? meds + unk allergy Pt. wound dressed + c-spined + boarded

Advanced Life Support

Time	Medication	Rate/Dose	Route
/	/	/	
/	/	/	
/	/	/	
/	/	/	
/	/	/	
/	/	/	
/	/	/	

Total Fluid Infused: _____ mls

DEFIB: Time:	Time:	Time:	Time:
Joules:	Joules:	Joules:	Joules:

Medical Control: ❏ Direct ❏ C-MED Channel _____
MD# _____   Hospital _____
Hospital Notified Enroute: ❏ Yes ❏ No
❏ C-MED ❏ Dispatcher

Other Response Units/Agencies:
Police/Fire/Paramedics

Unit # A65   EMT/Paramedic Signatures:
M. Fletcher #360   P. Masson #385   #

E.M.S. TRAINING PROGRAM
PATIENT CARE REPORT FORM

© 1992 Kennedy Associates

Patient Name: John Porter	Trip #: 012 / Date: 09·30·92
Address: 160 Park Ave	M.R.#: / Day: Wednesday
Boston MA	Dispatch To: / For: female fell
DOB: 08-18-20 Tel. #: 555-3213	210 main St West
Next of Kin:	Dispatch Time: 1332 / Arrival Time:
Address:	To Hospital: / At Hospital:
	Location at Dispatch: Community Hospital
Relationship: Tel. #:	Billing Information (circle):
Transported to: Transport Priority:	(Medicare) Medicaid BC/BS
Miles from: To:	Indust. Acc. Self Other
❏ No Transport	Subscriber:
REASON:	
	Policy #:

Physical Exam

Eye Opening: ☑ Spontaneous ❏ To Pain ❏ To Voice ❏ None

Verbal Response: ☑ Oriented ❏ Confused ❏ Inappropriate ❏ Incomprehensible ❏ None

Motor Response: ☑ Obedience ❏ Purposeful ❏ Withdrawal ❏ Flexion ❏ Extension ❏ None

Skin Condition: ☑ Normal ❏ Cool ❏ Hot ❏ Pale ❏ Flushed ❏ Cyanotic ❏ Diaphoretic

Vital Signs

❏ Unable to Obtain   ❏ Not attempted

REASON:

Time	BP	Pulse	Resp. Rate/Effort
13:42	208/P	84 R	18

Allergies: ☑ None / ❏ Unknown

Current Medications: Ativan/tylenol   ❏ None / ❏ Unknown

Brought with Pt.? ❏ Yes ❏ No

Suspected Diagnosis: ❏ Chronic ❏ Acute
❏ Major Trauma ❏ Acute Medical ❏ Cardiac Arrest ❏ Shock
❏ Minor Trauma ❏ Minor Medical ❏ Cardiac Disorder ❏ ETOH
☑ Soft Tissue Injury ❏ Burns ❏ Ortho ❏ OD/Poison
❏ Neuro ❏ Seizure ❏ Psych ❏ OB/GYN ❏ Neonate

Emergency Care: ❏ CPR ❏ Extricate ❏ Back/Neck Immobilize
☑ Bleed Control ☑ Bandage ❏ Splint ❏ Heat/Cold Applied
❏ O₂ Administration: _____ liters/minute via _____
Airway: ❏ Cleared ❏ Oral ❏ Nasal Size: _____ ❏ Suction
Intubate: ❏ Endotracheal ❏ Nasctracheal Size: _____
Assist Ventilation: Rate: _____ Method: _____
❏ ECG Monitor ❏ Rhythm Strip Attached
Transport Position: Sitting c̄ belt

Chief Complaint/History/Changes in Patient Status

LAC (L) HEAD
72 y.o. ♀ found sitting in bookstore
c̄ LAC Approx ½" (L) Temporal
Ø hemmorrhage. Pt sts she tripped
on sidewalk Ø L.O.C. Pt denies
neck/back pain. Pt c/o h/A
Uknown last tetanus
PE - A, O x3 Ø diaph skin w/d
HEENT⊖ pupil ⊖ reactive
B.S. clear/Equal Abd ⊖
Extremities ⊖ Back ⊖
PMH - HTN
med - Ativan, tylenol
All - NKDA
Tx - D, S, D bandage
Transport c̄ Δ To Hospital

Advanced Life Support

Time	/	Medication	/	Rate/Dose	/	Route
	/		/		/	
	/		/		/	
	/		/		/	
	/		/		/	
	/		/		/	
	/		/		/	
	/		/		/	

Total Fluid Infused: _____ mls

DEFIB: Time:	Time:	Time:	Time:
Joules:	Joules:	Joules:	Joules:

Medical Control: ❏ Direct ☑ C-MED Channel 3
MD# _____ Hospital _____
Hospital Notified Enroute: ☑ Yes ❏ No
☑ C-MED ❏ Dispatcher

Other Response Units/Agencies: Police

Unit # | EMT/Paramedic Signatures:
_____ # _____   _____ # _____   _____ # _____

E.M.S. TRAINING PROGRAM
PATIENT CARE REPORT FORM

© 1992 Kennedy Associates

Patient Name: Harriet Stevens	Trip #: 013 · Date: 9/30/92
Address: 46 Englewood Ave · Newton MA	M.R.#: · Day: Wed
	Dispatch To: · For: Respiratory Distress
DOB: 9-10-40 · Tel. #: 555-1462	Community Health Clinic
Next of Kin: Philip Stevens	Dispatch Time: 1035 · Arrival Time: 1045
Address: Same	To Hospital: 1056 · At Hospital: 1102
	Location at Dispatch:
Relationship: Husband · Tel. #: Same	Billing Information (circle):
Transported to: · Transport Priority:	Medicare (Medicaid) BC/BS
Miles from: · To:	Indust. Acc. Self Other
❑ No Transport · REASON:	Subscriber: Philip Stevens
	Policy #:

Physical Exam

Eye Opening: ☒ Spontaneous ❑ To Pain ❑ To Voice ❑ None

Verbal Response: ☒ Oriented ❑ Confused ❑ Inappropriate ❑ Incomprehensible ❑ None

Motor Response: ☒ Obedience ❑ Purposeful ❑ Withdrawal ❑ Flexion ❑ Extension ❑ None

Skin Condition: ☒ Normal ❑ Cool ❑ Hot ❑ Pale ❑ Flushed ❑ Cyanotic ❑ Diaphoretic

Chief Complaint/History/Changes in Patient Status

52 y o ♀ Difficulty breathing
Presents supine on clinic bed c̄ O₂ via n/c.
Clinic staff relates pt. was seated in
waiting room, started shaking & hyperventilat.
Through interpreter pt. relates ∅ complaints
(PE) Pt. CAOx3 skin w/Dc̄ good color abd
soft nontender good ROM.
(Tx) - semi-fowler to hosp ∅ Δ enroute.
(hx) - CHF (Rx) - Prozac (Allg) - unknown

Vital Signs

❑ Unable to Obtain   ❑ Not attempted

REASON:

Time	BP	Pulse	Resp. Rate/Effort
1048	140/76	76 R	16 n

Allergies: ❑ None ☒ Unknown

Current Medications: Listed ↗ ❑ None ❑ Unknown

Brought with Pt.? ❑ Yes ❑ No

Suspected Diagnosis: ❑ Chronic ❑ Acute
❑ Major Trauma ❑ Acute Medical ❑ Cardiac Arrest ❑ Shock
❑ Minor Trauma ❑ Minor Medical ❑ Cardiac Disorder ❑ ETOH
❑ Soft Tissue Injury ❑ Burns ❑ Ortho ❑ OD/Poison
❑ Neuro ❑ Seizure ❑ Psych ❑ OB/GYN ❑ Neonate

Advanced Life Support

Time /	Medication /	Rate/Dose /	Route
/	/	/	
/	/	/	
/	/	/	
/	/	/	
/	/	/	
/	/	/	
/	/	/	

Total Fluid Infused: _____ mls

Emergency Care: ❑ CPR ❑ Extricate ❑ Back/Neck Immobilize
❑ Bleed Control ❑ Bandage ❑ Splint ❑ Heat/Cold Applied
❑ O₂ Administration: _____ liters/minute via _____
Airway: ❑ Cleared ❑ Oral ❑ Nasal Size: _____ ❑ Suction
Intubate: ❑ Endotracheal ❑ Nasotracheal Size: _____
Assist Ventilation: Rate: _____ Method: _____
❑ ECG Monitor ❑ Rhythm Strip Attached
Transport Position: Semi-fowler

DEFIB: Time:	Time:	Time:	Time:
Joules:	Joules:	Joules:	Joules:

Medical Control: ❑ Direct ❑ C-MED Channel _____
MD# _____ Hospital _____
Hospital Notified Enroute: ❑ Yes ☒ No
❑ C-MED ❑ Dispatcher

Other Response Units/Agencies: _____

Unit # A28   EMT/Paramedic Signatures:
_____ # _____ # _____ #

E.M.S. TRAINING PROGRAM
PATIENT CARE REPORT FORM

© 1992 Kennedy Associat[e]

Patient Name: Paul Willard	Trip #: 014　　Date: 9/30/92
Address: 850 Revere Ave　Somerville MA	M.R.#:　　Day: Wednesday / MVA
DOB: 5-18-72　Tel. #: 555-1273	Dispatch To: River St at Oak Sq　For:
Next of Kin: Peter Willard	Dispatch Time:　Arrival Time:
Address: S/A	To Hospital:　At Hospital:
	Location at Dispatch:
Relationship: Father　Tel. #:	Billing Information (circle):
Transported to: T.G.H.　Transport Priority: 2	Medicare　Medicaid　BC/BS
Miles from:　To:	Indust. Acc.　(Self)　Other
❑ No Transport　REASON:	Subscriber:
	Policy #:

Physical Exam

Eye Opening
- ☑ Spontaneous ❑ To Pain
- ❑ To Voice ❑ None

Verbal Response
- ☑ Oriented ❑ Confused
- ❑ Inappropriate ❑ Incomprehensible ❑ None

Motor Response
- ☑ Obedience ❑ Purposeful ❑ Withdrawal
- ❑ Flexion ❑ Extension ❑ None

Skin Condition
- ☑ Normal ❑ Cool ❑ Hot ❑ Pale
- ❑ Flushed ❑ Cyanotic ❑ Diaphoretic

Vital Signs

❑ Unable to Obtain　❑ Not attempted
REASON:

Time	BP	Pulse	Resp. Rate/Effort
	132/88	88	16

Allergies: NKDA　❑ None ❑ Unknown

Current Medications:　☑ None ❑ Unknown

Brought with Pt.?　❑ Yes ❑ No

Suspected Diagnosis: ❑ Chronic ❑ Acute
- ❑ Major Trauma ❑ Acute Medical ❑ Cardiac Arrest ❑ Shock
- ❑ Minor Trauma ❑ Minor Medical ❑ Cardiac Disorder ❑ ETOH
- ❑ Soft Tissue Injury ❑ Burns ☑ Ortho ❑ OD/Poison
- ❑ Neuro ❑ Seizure ❑ Psych ❑ OB/GYN ❑ Neonate

Emergency Care: ❑ CPR ❑ Extricate ☑ Back/Neck Immobilize
❑ Bleed Control ❑ Bandage ☑ Splint ☑ Heat (Cold Applied)
❑ O₂ Administration: _____ liters/minute via _____
Airway: ❑ Cleared ❑ Oral ❑ Nasal Size: _____ ❑ Suction
Intubate: ❑ Endotracheal ❑ Nasotracheal Size: _____
Assist Ventilation: Rate: _____ Method: _____
❑ ECG Monitor ❑ Rhythm Strip Attached
Transport Position: C-Spined

Unit # A33　EMT/Paramedic Signatures: Jim Prince # 376　Nancy Rush # 389　_____ # ____

Chief Complaint/History/Changes in Patient Status

20yo ♂ found in the back seat of a car on its roof post MVA car was struck then rolled over into parked car ∅ seatbelt denies striking his head or loc. Heavey damage ¥/o left wrist pain.
PMH: ∅ Med: ∅ Aller: NKDA
PE: 20yo ♂ CAX3 oriented to Day, Date, Place, self, ∅ lac's or swelling to his head, ENT clear pupils 6mm perrl, ∅ deform or tenderness to neck or back. Trach midline ∅ JVD chest rize equal ∅ cp BBS = clear Abd soft not tender, pelvis sturdy lower extremities ∅ deform Full range of motion, tenderness left wrist ∅ deform/swell reduced range of motion
Pt C-spined trans to hospital

Advanced Life Support

Time	/	Medication	/	Rate/Dose	/	Route
	/		/		/	
	/		/		/	
	/		/		/	
	/		/		/	
	/		/		/	
	/		/		/	

Total Fluid Infused: _____ mls

DEFIB: Time:	Time:	Time:	Time:
Joules:	Joules:	Joules:	Joules:

Medical Control: ❑ Direct ❑ C-MED Channel _____
MD# _____　Hospital _____
Hospital Notified Enroute:　❑ Yes ❑ No
❑ C-MED ❑ Dispatcher

Other Response Units/Agencies: Police / Fire / Paramedics

E.M.S. TRAINING PROGRAM
PATIENT CARE REPORT FORM

© 1992 Kennedy Associates

Patient Name: John Hines	Trip #: 015 — Date: 9-30-92
Address: 45 Garden St	M.R.#: — Day: W
Chelsea MA	Dispatch To: — For: Injury
DOB: 3-16-05 Tel. #: 555-7245	Gourmet Deli /118 Broad St
Next of Kin: Mildred Hines	Dispatch Time: 1220 — Arrival Time: 1226
Address: Same	To Hospital: — At Hospital: 1240

Location at Dispatch:

Relationship: Sister Tel. #:

Transported to: Community Hosp. Transport Priority:

Miles from: To:

❑ No Transport
REASON:

Billing Information (circle): (**Medicare**) Medicaid BC/BS
Indust. Acc. Self Other

Subscriber:

Policy #:

Physical Exam

Eye Opening: ☑ Spontaneous ❑ To Pain ❑ To Voice ❑ None

Verbal Response: ☑ Oriented ❑ Confused ❑ Inappropriate ❑ Incomprehensible ❑ None

Motor Response: ☑ Obedience ❑ Purposeful ❑ Withdrawal ❑ Flexion ❑ Extension ❑ None

Skin Condition: ☑ Normal ❑ Cool ❑ Hot ❑ Pale ❑ Flushed ❑ Cyanotic ❑ Diaphoretic

Vital Signs

❑ Unable to Obtain ❑ Not attempted
REASON:

Time	BP	Pulse	Resp. Rate/Effort
1228 ♀	160/100	64 R	12 ∩
1232 ♀	150/96	60 R	12 ∩

Chief Complaint/History/Changes in Patient Status

(HPI) 87 yo ♂ found seated on chair in restaraunt c/o facial injury after fall down 3 steps. Pt. relates slipping & landing prone on floor. ∅ loc ∅ neck. c/p or back pn

(PE) Pt CAOX3 skin W/D c̄ good color PEARL X 3mm. minor abrasion to ® temporal region c̄ ∅ bleeding. Minor abrasion to upper lip c̄ ∅ bleeding minor abrasion to Ⓛ wrist c̄ ∅ bleeding Good CSM

(TX) - absence of thyroid, middle ear problem ® - Sinthroid Sinequan

(Allg) NKDA

Allergies: NKDA ❑ None ❑ Unknown

Current Medications: ❑ None ❑ Unknown

Brought with Pt.? ❑ Yes ❑ No

Suspected Diagnosis: ❑ Chronic ❑ Acute
❑ Major Trauma ❑ Acute Medical ❑ Cardiac Arrest ❑ Shock
❑ Minor Trauma ❑ Minor Medical ❑ Cardiac Disorder ❑ ETOH
❑ Soft Tissue Injury ❑ Burns ❑ Ortho ❑ OD/Poison
❑ Neuro ❑ Seizure ❑ Psych ❑ OB/GYN ❑ Neonate

Advanced Life Support

Time	/	Medication	/	Rate/Dose	/	Route
	/		/		/	
	/		/		/	
	/		/		/	
	/		/		/	
	/		/		/	
	/		/		/	
	/		/		/	

Total Fluid Infused: mls

Emergency Care: ❑ CPR ❑ Extricate ❑ Back/Neck Immobilize
❑ Bleed Control ❑ Bandage ❑ Splint ❑ Heat/Cold Applied
❑ O₂ Administration: _____ liters/minute via _____
Airway: ❑ Cleared ❑ Oral ❑ Nasal Size: _____ ❑ Suction
Intubate: ❑ Endotracheal ❑ Nasotracheal Size: _____
Assist Ventilation: Rate: _____ Method: _____
❑ ECG Monitor ❑ Rhythm Strip Attached
Transport Position: Seated

DEFIB: Time:	Time:	Time:	Time:
Joules:	Joules:	Joules:	Joules:

Medical Control: ❑ Direct ❑ C-MED Channel _____
MD#_____ Hospital _____
Hospital Notified Enroute: ❑ Yes ☑ No
❑ C-MED ❑ Dispatcher

Other Response Units/Agencies:

Unit # EMT/Paramedic Signatures:
David Ross # 316 Bill Welch # _____ # _____

E.M.S. TRAINING PROGRAM
PATIENT CARE REPORT FORM

© 1992 Kennedy Associates

Patient Name: John McGrath	Trip #: 016 Date: 9/30/1992
Address:	M.R.#: Day: Wed.
	Dispatch To: For: Injury
DOB: Tel. #:	600 Wash St. outside
Next of Kin:	Dispatch Time: Arrival Time:
Address:	To Hospital: At Hospital:
	Location at Dispatch:
Relationship: Tel. #:	Billing Information (circle):
Transported to: Transport Priority:	Medicare Medicaid BC/BS
Miles from: To:	Indust. Acc. Self Other
❏ No Transport	Subscriber:
REASON:	
	Policy #:

Physical Exam

Eye Opening: ☑ Spontaneous ❏ To Pain ❏ To Voice ❏ None

Verbal Response: ☑ Oriented ❏ Confused ❏ Inappropriate ❏ Incomprehensible ❏ None

Motor Response: ☑ Obedience ❏ Purposeful ❏ Withdrawal ❏ Flexion ❏ Extension ❏ None

Skin Condition: ☑ Normal ❏ Cool ❏ Hot ❏ Pale ❏ Flushed ❏ Cyanotic ❏ Diaphoretic

Vital Signs

❏ Unable to Obtain   ❏ Not attempted
REASON:

Time	BP	Pulse	Resp. Rate/Effort

Allergies: NKDA   ☑ None ❏ Unknown

Current Medications: ☑ None ❏ Unknown

Brought with Pt.? ❏ Yes ❏ No

Suspected Diagnosis: ❏ Chronic ❏ Acute
❏ Major Trauma ❏ Acute Medical ❏ Cardiac Arrest ❏ Shock
❏ Minor Trauma ❏ Minor Medical ❏ Cardiac Disorder ❏ ETOH
❏ Soft Tissue Injury ❏ Burns ❏ Ortho ❏ OD/Poison
❏ Neuro ❏ Seizure ❏ Psych ❏ OB/GYN ❏ Neonate

Chief Complaint/History/Changes in Patient Status

21 yo ♂ ? Dislocated ® Shoulder
HPI: Pt reports he was pushed to the ground causing him to land on his ® anterior lateral Shoulder. Now c/o severe discomfort & inability to move arm.
PE: CAOx3 21 y/o ♂ seated on ground c̄ his ® arm flexed @ the level of his shoulder ⊕ cap ill refill & grasp. No H/N/B pain. No other complaints at this time
PMH → meds → Allg → denies all

Splinted in position found Ice Applied Ø Δ → Hospital

Advanced Life Support

Time	/	Medication	/	Rate/Dose	/	Route
	/		/		/	
	/		/		/	
	/		/		/	
	/		/		/	
	/		/		/	
	/		/		/	

Total Fluid Infused: mls

Emergency Care: ❏ CPR ❏ Extricate ❏ Back/Neck Immobilize
❏ Bleed Control ❏ Bandage ❏ Splint ❏ Heat/Cold Applied
❏ O₂ Administration: _____ liters/minute via _____
Airway: ❏ Cleared ❏ Oral ❏ Nasal Size: _____ ❏ Suction
Intubate: ❏ Endotracheal ❏ Nasotracheal Size: _____
Assist Ventilation: Rate: _____ Method: _____
❏ ECG Monitor ❏ Rhythm Strip Attached
Transport Position: Seated

DEFIB: Time:	Time:	Time:	Time:
Joules:	Joules:	Joules:	Joules:

Medical Control: ❏ Direct ❏ C-MED Channel _____
MD#_____ Hospital _____
Hospital Notified Enroute: ❏ Yes ❏ No
❏ C-MED ❏ Dispatcher

Other Response Units/Agencies: Police

Unit # A46   EMT/Paramedic Signatures: Joe Jase # _____   # _____   # _____

E.M.S. TRAINING PROGRAM
PATIENT CARE REPORT FORM

© 1992 Kennedy Associates

Patient Name: Suzanne Platt	Trip #: 017 Date: Sept. 30, 1992
Address: 19 Parsons way	M.R.#: Day: Thursday
Hyde Park MB	Dispatch To: For: Illness
DOB: Jan. 22, 1921 Tel. #: 555-4213	19 Parsons way
Next of Kin:	Dispatch Time: 1208 Arrival Time:
Address:	To Hospital: At Hospital:
	Location at Dispatch:
Relationship: Tel. #:	Billing Information (circle):
Transported to: C.H. Transport Priority: 2	Medicare Medicaid BC/BS
Miles from: To:	Indust. Acc. Self Other
❑ No Transport REASON:	Subscriber:
	Policy #:

Physical Exam

Eye Opening: ☒ Spontaneous ❑ To Pain ❑ To Voice ❑ None

Verbal Response: ☒ Oriented ❑ Confused ❑ Inappropriate ❑ Incomprehensible ❑ None

Motor Response: ☒ Obedience ❑ Purposeful ❑ Withdrawal ❑ Flexion ❑ Extension ❑ None

Skin Condition: ☒ Normal ❑ Cool ❑ Hot ❑ Pale ❑ Flushed ❑ Cyanotic ❑ Diaphoretic

Vital Signs

❑ Unable to Obtain   ❑ Not attempted
REASON:

Time	BP	Pulse	Resp. Rate/Effort
1220	130/60	62	18

Allergies: PCN Percodan   ❑ None   ❑ Unknown

Current Medications: See ⟶   ❑ None   ❑ Unknown

Brought with Pt.?   ❑ Yes   ❑ No

Suspected Diagnosis: ❑ Chronic   ❑ Acute
❑ Major Trauma ❑ Acute Medical ❑ Cardiac Arrest ❑ Shock
❑ Minor Trauma ❑ Minor Medical ❑ Cardiac Disorder ❑ ETOH
❑ Soft Tissue Injury ❑ Burns ❑ Ortho ❑ OD/Poison
❑ Neuro ❑ Seizure ❑ Psych ❑ OB/GYN ❑ Neonate

Emergency Care: ❑ CPR ❑ Extricate ❑ Back/Neck Immobilize
❑ Bleed Control ❑ Bandage ❑ Splint ❑ Heat/Cold Applied
❑ O₂ Administration: _____ liters/minute via _____
Airway: ❑ Cleared ❑ Oral ❑ Nasal Size: _____ ❑ Suction
Intubate: ❑ Endotracheal ❑ Nasotracheal Size: _____
Assist Ventilation: Rate: _____ Method: _____
❑ ECG Monitor ❑ Rhythm Strip Attached
Transport Position: Semi-fowles

Unit # A55   EMT/Paramedic Signatures: Christine Reary #348   F.A. #365   #

Chief Complaint/History/Changes in Patient Status

Blood clot ⓛ foot/leg
71yo ♀ found supine @ place of residence ē VNA
on scene VNA states questioning blood clot ⓛ
foot/leg (pain began Sunday) UTI infection
↓ coumadin level 12.6. VNA informed pt. MD and
wished to have pt. evaluated pt states she has
throbbing pain in ⓛ foot travelling up to groin
"pain so intense keep pt up all evening
PE of found pt to be CAOx3 ABC's intact HEENT
unremarkable PERL denies N/V/D ⊖ JVD chest
unremarkable ⊖ CP lungs clear ⓛ bilaterally ABD
soft nontender x4 quads. pt is stating she has some
mild ↓ back pain ⊖ trauma) no deformities ℞EXTREM.
unremarkable ē pulses/neurological function/range
of motion ↓ Extremities Note purple coloring of ⓛ
extremity ē pulses present ē adequate neurological
function. vital signs BP 130/60 P62 R18 all else
unremarkable pt is stable.   Tx of pt. includes
elevation ↓ extremity Transport and monitor
while enroute No change in transport

Advanced Life Support

Time	Medication	Rate/Dose	Route
Past medical Hx - IDDM CAD CHF S/P bypass			
Surgery			
Medications ē NITRO, KCL, colace Zaditylen			
Insulin lopressor Cardizem			
Isordil xanax Bumex Doxepin			
	/	/	/
	/	/	/
	/	/	/

Total Fluid Infused: _____ mls

DEFIB: Time: _____ Time: _____ Time: _____ Time: _____
Joules: _____ Joules: _____ Joules: _____ Joules: _____

Medical Control: ❑ Direct ❑ C-MED Channel _____
MD# _____ Hospital _____
Hospital Notified Enroute: ❑ Yes ❑ No
❑ C-MED ❑ Dispatcher

Other Response Units/Agencies:

E.M.S. TRAINING PROGRAM
PATIENT CARE REPORT FORM

© 1992 Kennedy Associate

Patient Name: Karen Thomsen	Trip #: 018	Date: September 30, 19
Address: 56 Burr Ave	M.R.#:	Day: Wednesday
Everett MA	Dispatch To:	For: MVA
DOB: March 29, 1969 Tel. #: 555-6437	60 Hamilton ST	
Next of Kin: John Thomsen	Dispatch Time: 0941	Arrival Time: 0944
Address: S/A	To Hospital: 0952	At Hospital: 0959

Location at Dispatch: 4th ST / 6th Ave

Relationship: Husband Tel. #: Same	Billing Information (circle):
Transported to: Comm. Hosp. Transport Priority:	Medicare Medicaid (BC/BS)
Miles from: To: 3	Indust. Acc. Self Other
❏ No Transport	Subscriber: Patient
REASON:	Group plan People's Investment Bank
	Policy #: not available

Physical Exam

Eye Opening: ☒ Spontaneous ❏ To Pain ❏ To Voice ❏ None

Verbal Response: ☒ Oriented ❏ Confused ❏ Inappropriate ❏ Incomprehensible ❏ None

Motor Response: ☒ Obedience ❏ Purposeful ❏ Withdrawal ❏ Flexion ❏ Extension ❏ None

Skin Condition: ☒ Normal ❏ Cool ❏ Hot ❏ Pale ❏ Flushed ❏ Cyanotic ❏ Diaphoretic

Vital Signs

❏ Unable to Obtain   ❏ Not attempted
REASON:

Time	BP	Pulse	Resp. Rate/Effort
0950	142/70	88 Reg 2+	16 Normal/Full

Allergies: NKA   ☒ None ❏ Unknown

Current Medications: ☒ None ❏ Unknown

Brought with Pt.? ❏ Yes ❏ No

Suspected Diagnosis: ❏ Chronic ☒ Acute
❏ Major Trauma ❏ Acute Medical ❏ Cardiac Arrest ❏ Shock
❏ Minor Trauma ❏ Minor Medical ❏ Cardiac Disorder ❏ ETOH
☒ Soft Tissue Injury ❏ Burns ❏ Ortho ❏ OD/Poison
❏ Neuro ❏ Seizure ❏ Psych ❏ OB/GYN ❏ Neonate

Emergency Care: ❏ CPR ❏ Extricate ❏ Back/Neck Immobilize
☒ Bleed Control ☒ Bandage ☒ Splint ❏ Heat/Cold Applied
❏ O2 Administration: _____ liters/minute via _____
Airway: ❏ Cleared ❏ Oral ❏ Nasal Size: _____ ❏ Suction
Intubate: ❏ Endotracheal ❏ Nasotracheal Size: _____
Assist Ventilation: Rate: _____ Method: _____
❏ ECG Monitor ❏ Rhythm Strip Attached
Transport Position: Seated

Chief Complaint/History/Changes in Patient Status

(HPI) 23 yo ♀ found seated in police car c/o minor abrasions to (L) arm c̄ pain p̄ being struck from behind (L side) by a bicycle messenger. Pt. relates falling forward and guarding fall c̄ arms & landing on her travel bag. No loss of consciousne No pain at head, neck, back or chest.

(PMH) No hx of medical disorders

(meds) No Rx meds taken (NKA)

(PE) alert and oriented, skin warm and dry good color pupils =/react to light. Swollen (L) maxillary region. Minor abrasions to (R) & (L) elbows c̄ slight bleeding. Abd - has aprox 4" abrasion to upper abd not bleeding. (R) knee has minor abrasion not bleeding.

(Tx) Dress and bandage abrasions sling and swathe (L) arm. Transport to Hospital. Remains stable during Transport

Advanced Life Support

Time	/	Medication	/	Rate/Dose	/	Route
	/		/		/	
	/		/		/	
	/		/		/	
	/		/		/	
	/		/		/	
	/		/		/	

Total Fluid Infused: _____ mls

DEFIB: Time:	Time:	Time:	Time:
Joules:	Joules:	Joules:	Joules:

Medical Control: ❏ Direct ❏ C-MED Channel _____
MD# _____ Hospital _____
Hospital Notified Enroute: ❏ Yes ❏ No
❏ C-MED ❏ Dispatcher

Other Response Units/Agencies:

Unit # A26   EMT/Paramedic Signatures: Gwen Merritt #359   Donna Newton #366 #_____

E.M.S. TRAINING PROGRAM
PATIENT CARE REPORT FORM

© 1992 Kennedy Associates

Patient Name: James Tucker	Trip #: 019 · Date: Sept 30 '92
Address: 38 Edwards St · Brookline MA	M.R.#: 200 40 60 5 · Day: Wed.
DOB: · Tel. #:	Dispatch To: 46 Mason Rd · For: Injury
Next of Kin: Susan	Dispatch Time: 0611 · Arrival Time: 0617
Address:	To Hospital: · At Hospital:
	Location at Dispatch: Border Square
Relationship: Wife · Tel. #:	Billing Information (circle):
Transported to: TGH · Transport Priority: 3	Medicare Medicaid BC/BS
Miles from: · To:	(Indust. Acc.) Self Other
☐ No Transport REASON:	Subscriber: J+B Construction 409 Washington St Arlington
	Policy #:

Physical Exam

Eye Opening	☒ Spontaneous ☐ To Pain / ☐ To Voice ☐ None
Verbal Response	☒ Oriented ☐ Confused / ☐ Inappropriate ☐ Incomprehensible ☐ None
Motor Response	☒ Obedience ☐ Purposeful ☐ Withdrawal / ☐ Flexion ☐ Extension ☐ None
Skin Condition	☒ Normal ☐ Cool ☐ Hot ☐ Pale / ☐ Flushed ☐ Cyanotic ☐ Diaphoretic

Vital Signs

☐ Unable to Obtain   ☐ Not attempted
REASON:

Time	BP	Pulse	Resp. Rate/Effort
0620	186/100	88	16

Allergies: ☒ None ☐ Unknown

Current Medications: BLOCADREN   ☐ None ☐ Unknown

Brought with Pt.? ☐ Yes ☐ No

Suspected Diagnosis: ☐ Chronic ☐ Acute
☒ Major Trauma ☐ Acute Medical ☐ Cardiac Arrest ☐ Shock
☒ Minor Trauma ☐ Minor Medical ☐ Cardiac Disorder ☐ ETOH
☐ Soft Tissue Injury ☐ Burns ☒ Ortho? ☐ OD/Poison
☐ Neuro ☐ Seizure ☐ Psych ☐ OB/GYN ☐ Neonate

Emergency Care: ☐ CPR ☐ Extricate ☐ Back/Neck Immobilize
☐ Bleed Control ☐ Bandage ☒ Splint ☒ Heat (Cold Applied)
☐ O₂ Administration: _____ liters/minute via _____
Airway: ☐ Cleared ☐ Oral ☐ Nasal Size: _____ ☐ Suction
Intubate: ☐ Endotracheal ☐ Nasotracheal Size: _____
Assist Ventilation: Rate: _____ Method: _____
☐ ECG Monitor ☐ Rhythm Strip Attached
Transport Position: SEATED

Unit # A59   EMT/Paramedic Signatures: Karl Loring #346 S.H. #_____   #_____

Chief Complaint/History/Changes in Patient Status

(R) leg injury
40 Y.O. ♂ c/o pain to (R) CALF AFTER EXERTION ON PUSHING HEAVY OBJECT & OVERFLEXION OF (R) FOOT. PT. DENIES TWISTING OR ROTATING MVMT BUT FELT "POP" AT TIME OF INJ. PT. DENIES TINGLING OR NUMBNESS DENIES RADIATION TO UPPER LEG. PT. AMBULATORY BUT c/o PAIN ON BEARING DOWN c WT ON (R) FOOT. DENIES PAIN TO KNEE OR FOOT.
(PE) C/A/0X3, NAD, SKIN WARM/ DRY. PERRL @ 4mm. LUNGS CLEAR ABD SOFT/NONTENDER GOOD ROM All EXTREM INC (R) FOOT. GOOD DISTAL PULSES & CSM (R) FOOT NO SWELLING OR ECCYMOSIS EVIDENT 2° OTHERWISE BENIGN
(PMH) HTN (MED) BLOCADREN (ALL) Ø

Advanced Life Support

Time	/ Medication	/ Rate/Dose	/ Route
(Tx)	SPLINT, ICE & TRANSPORT		
	/	/	/
	/	/	/
	/	/	/
	/	/	/
	/	/	/
	/	/	/
	/	/	/

Total Fluid Infused: _____ mls

DEFIB: Time:	Time:	Time:	Time:
Joules:	Joules:	Joules:	Joules:

Medical Control: ☐ Direct ☐ C-MED Channel _____
MD#_____ Hospital _____
Hospital Notified Enroute: ☐ Yes ☒ No
☐ C-MED ☐ Dispatcher

Other Response Units/Agencies: Fire

E.M.S. TRAINING PROGRAM
PATIENT CARE REPORT FORM

© 1992 Kennedy Associates

Patient Name: Frank True	Trip #: 020 Date: 09/30/92
Address: 48 Jepson Blvd	M.R.#: Day: Wednsdy
Jamaica Plain MA	person shot
DOB: 06/08/42 Tel. #: 555-6675	Dispatch To: For:
	48 Jepson Blvd #2110
Next of Kin:	Dispatch Time: Arrival Time:
Address:	To Hospital: At Hospital:
	Location at Dispatch:
Relationship: Tel. #:	Billing Information (circle):
Transported to: C.H. Transport Priority: 3	Medicare Medicaid BC/BS
Miles from: To:	Indust. Acc. (Self) Other
❑ No Transport	Subscriber:
REASON:	
	Policy #:

Physical Exam

Eye Opening: ☑ Spontaneous ❑ To Pain ❑ To Voice ❑ None

Verbal Response: ☑ Oriented ❑ Confused ❑ Inappropriate ❑ Incomprehensible ❑ None

Motor Response: ☑ Obedience ❑ Purposeful ❑ Withdrawal ❑ Flexion ❑ Extension ❑ None

Skin Condition: ☑ Normal ❑ Cool ❑ Hot ❑ Pale ❑ Flushed ❑ Cyanotic ❑ Diaphoretic

Vital Signs

❑ Unable to Obtain   ❑ Not attempted
REASON:

Time	BP	Pulse	Resp. Rate/Effort
	150/102	108	18/normal

Allergies: ☑ None ❑ Unknown

Current Medications: ☑ None ❑ Unknown

Brought with Pt.? ❑ Yes ❑ No

Suspected Diagnosis: ❑ Chronic ❑ Acute
❑ Major Trauma ❑ Acute Medical ❑ Cardiac Arrest ❑ Shock
❑ Minor Trauma ❑ Minor Medical ❑ Cardiac Disorder ❑ ETOH
❑ Soft Tissue Injury ❑ Burns ❑ Ortho ❑ OD/Poison
❑ Neuro ❑ Seizure ❑ Psych ❑ OB/GYN ❑ Neonate

Emergency Care: ❑ CPR ❑ Extricate ❑ Back/Neck Immobilize
❑ Bleed Control ☑ Bandage ❑ Splint ❑ Heat/Cold Applied
❑ O₂ Administration: _____ liters/minute via _____
Airway: ❑ Cleared ❑ Oral ❑ Nasal Size: _____ ❑ Suction
Intubate: ❑ Endotracheal ❑ Nasotracheal Size: _____
Assist Ventilation: Rate: _____ Method: _____
❑ ECG Monitor ❑ Rhythm Strip Attached
Transport Position: Seated

Chief Complaint/History/Changes in Patient Status

50 yo ♂ hx of old G.S.W. = 20 years ago, found walking to ambulance s/o ⓛ leg pain ? infection Admits to using heavy E.T.O.H. difficult to obtain complete history. Denies fever chills N+V. Last drink 20 minutes ago. Past history as above meds none P. eval. Conscious oriented skin warm ⓛ leg - old injury has Newly opened area inflammed with odor

Pt. given 4x4, elevation transport to Hospital

Advanced Life Support

Time /	Medication /	Rate/Dose /	Route
/	/	/	
/	/	/	
/	/	/	
/	/	/	
/	/	/	
/	/	/	
/	/	/	

Total Fluid Infused: _____ mls

DEFIB: Time:	Time:	Time:	Time:
Joules:	Joules:	Joules:	Joules:

Medical Control: ❑ Direct ❑ C-MED Channel _____
MD# _____ Hospital _____
Hospital Notified Enroute: ❑ Yes ❑ No
❑ C-MED ❑ Dispatcher

Other Response Units/Agencies:

Unit #	EMT/Paramedic Signatures:
	_____ # _____ _____ # _____ _____ # _____

E.M.S. TRAINING PROGRAM
PATIENT CARE REPORT FORM

© 1992 Kennedy Associates

Patient Name: John Moore	Trip #: 021 Date: 9/30/92
Address: 68 High St	M.R.#: Day: Wed.
Boston MA	Dispatch To: For: Injury
DOB: 5-5-20 Tel. #: 555-1682	68 High St
Next of Kin: Pauline	Dispatch Time: 0025 Arrival Time: 0030
Address: Same	To Hospital: 0041 At Hospital: 0051
	Location at Dispatch: Satelite Station

Relationship: wife   Tel. #: 555-1682
Transported to: T.G.H.   Transport Priority: 3
Miles from: To:
☐ No Transport
REASON:

Billing Information (circle): Medicare   Medicaid   (BC/BS)
Indust. Acc.   Self   Other
Subscriber: John Moore
Policy #:

Physical Exam

Eye Opening: ☒ Spontaneous   ☐ To Pain   ☐ To Voice   ☐ None

Verbal Response: ☒ Oriented   ☐ Confused   ☐ Inappropriate   ☐ Incomprehensible   ☐ None

Motor Response: ☒ Obedience   ☐ Purposeful   ☐ Withdrawal   ☐ Flexion   ☐ Extension   ☐ None

Skin Condition: ☒ Normal   ☐ Cool   ☐ Hot   ☐ Pale   ☐ Flushed   ☐ Cyanotic   ☐ Diaphoretic

Vital Signs

☐ Unable to Obtain   ☐ Not attempted
REASON:

Time	BP	Pulse	Resp. Rate/Effort
0035	158/90	100	

Allergies: ☐ None   ☐ Unknown

Current Medications: ☐ None   ☐ Unknown

See (R) →

Brought with Pt.?   ☐ Yes   ☐ No

Suspected Diagnosis: ☐ Chronic   ☐ Acute
☐ Major Trauma   ☐ Acute Medical   ☐ Cardiac Arrest   ☐ Shock
☒ Minor Trauma   ☐ Minor Medical   ☐ Cardiac Disorder   ☐ ETOH
☐ Soft Tissue Injury   ☐ Burns   ☐ Ortho   ☐ OD/Poison
☐ Neuro   ☐ Seizure   ☐ Psych   ☐ OB/GYN   ☐ Neonate

Chief Complaint/History/Changes in Patient Status

(L) Shoulder Disloc.

(HPI) 72 yo ♂ ℅ (L) shoulder pn consistent to that of pn from Hx of shoulder dislocation Pt St he twisted shoulder while sleeping Pt found supine in bed

(PN) ∅ numbness/tingling denies any additional injuries or illness

(PE) Pt C/A ↓ Ox3 skin warm/dry ENT clear Head/chest palp intact ABD soft pedal symmetry Pt ambulatory on scene (L) shoulder presents c̄ mild anterior deformity ↑ pn on movement + palp ↓ ROM ∅ bruising - Good distal pulses + movement of fingers

(tx) PT transported c̄ Sling + swathe c̄ relief

(PmH) MI x 13 yrs
(meds) Isosorbide/Quinadine/Doxapin
(Allg) ∅

Advanced Life Support

Time /	Medication /	Rate/Dose /	Route
/	/	/	
/	/	/	
/	/	/	
/	/	/	
/	/	/	
/	/	/	
/	/	/	
/	/	/	

Total Fluid Infused: mls

Emergency Care: ☐ CPR   ☐ Extricate   ☐ Back/Neck Immobilize
☐ Bleed Control   ☐ Bandage   ☒ Splint   ☒ Heat/(Cold) Applied
☐ O₂ Administration: _____ liters/minute via _____
Airway: ☐ Cleared   ☐ Oral   ☐ Nasal Size: _____ ☐ Suction
Intubate: ☐ Endotracheal   ☐ Nasotracheal Size: _____
Assist Ventilation: Rate: _____ Method: _____
☐ ECG Monitor   ☐ Rhythm Strip Attached
Transport Position: Fowler

DEFIB: Time:	Time:	Time:	Time:
Joules:	Joules:	Joules:	Joules:

Medical Control: ☐ Direct   ☐ C-MED Channel _____
MD# _____ Hospital _____
Hospital Notified Enroute: ☐ Yes   ☐ No
☐ C-MED   ☐ Dispatcher

Other Response Units/Agencies:

Unit # A64   EMT/Paramedic Signatures: Kenneth Russell #382   Jan Victor #352   #

© 1992 Kennedy Associat[...]

E.M.S. TRAINING PROGRAM
PATIENT CARE REPORT FORM

Patient Name: Philip Lamb
Address: 894 Turnpike St
Worcester MA
DOB: 9-18-59   Tel. #: 555-4484
Next of Kin: Caroline Lamb
Address: Same
Relationship: Mother   Tel. #:
Transported to: T.G.H   Transport Priority: 3
Miles from: 396.4   To: 408.5
☐ No Transport
REASON:

Trip #: 022   Date: September 30 '9[...]
M.R.#:   Day: Wed.
Dispatch To: For: MVA
N. Market & S. main st?
Dispatch Time: Arrival Time:
To Hospital: At Hospital:
Location at Dispatch:
Billing Information (circle):
Medicare   Medicaid   BC/BS
Indust. Acc.   Self   Other
Subscriber:
Policy #:

Physical Exam

Eye Opening	☒ Spontaneous ☐ To Pain	
	☐ To Voice ☐ None	
Verbal Response	☒ Oriented ☐ Confused	
	☐ Inappropriate ☐ Incomprehensible ☐ None	
Motor Response	☒ Obedience ☐ Purposeful ☐ Withdrawal	
	☐ Flexion ☐ Extension ☐ None	
Skin Condition	☒ Normal ☐ Cool ☐ Hot ☐ Pale	
	☐ Flushed ☐ Cyanotic ☐ Diaphoretic	

Vital Signs

☐ Unable to Obtain   ☐ Not attempted
REASON:

Time	BP	Pulse	Resp. Rate/Effort
	150/86	118	16-20

Allergies: Ø   ☒ None   ☐ Unknown
Current Medications: Lithium   ☐ None   ☐ Unknown
Brought with Pt.?   ☐ Yes   ☐ No

Suspected Diagnosis: ☐ Chronic   ☐ Acute
☐ Major Trauma ☐ Acute Medical ☐ Cardiac Arrest ☐ Shock
☐ Minor Trauma ☐ Minor Medical ☐ Cardiac Disorder ☐ ETOH
☒ Soft Tissue Injury ☐ Burns ☐ Ortho ☐ OD/Poison
☐ Neuro ☐ Seizure ☐ Psych ☐ OB/GYN ☐ Neonate

Emergency Care: ☐ CPR ☐ Extricate ☒ Back/Neck Immobilize
☐ Bleed Control ☐ Bandage ☐ Splint ☐ Heat/Cold Applied
☐ O₂ Administration: _____ liters/minute via _____
Airway: ☐ Cleared ☐ Oral ☐ Nasal Size: _____ ☐ Suction
Intubate: ☐ Endotracheal ☐ Nasotracheal Size: _____
Assist Ventilation: Rate: _____ Method: _____
☐ ECG Monitor ☐ Rhythm Strip Attached
Transport Position: Supine long board
Unit # A40   EMT/Paramedic Signatures: J Heron #315   T-Garth #316

Chief Complaint/History/Changes in Patient Status

found 33 y.o. ♂ con't Alert sittin[g]
in rear of Police car p̄ an MVA
Ⓒ Ⓒ Ⓛ temperal area ½" Lac c̄
dizziness + neck, back pain.
(HPI) Pt's was involved in an head-o[n]
MVA. Pt was driving down the wrong
side of the road. Pt was restrained
Heavy frontend damage to Pt's car.
Windshield intact also the steering
wheel, unkn rate of speed
Pt stated he was uncon. for approx 5m[in]
Pt denies ETOH
(PMH) chemical imbalance, MED Lithium
NKDA
(PE) con't Alert + Ox3 P108 BP 150/86
Resp 16-20. Pupils 4mm E+R to ligh[t]
Skin W/D, color good cap. refill <2se[c]
(+) flexion/extension of all planters
Pt has a small lac to Ⓛ temperal
area of head - Pt c/o neck and lumba[r]
back pain

Advanced Life Support

Time	/	Medication	/	Rate/Dose	/	Route
(Tx)		c-spine Immobil., Trans s̄ Δ	/		/	
		/		/		
		/		/		
		/		/		
		/		/		
		/		/		
		/		/		

Total Fluid Infused: _____ mls

DEFIB:	Time:	Time:	Time:	Time:
	Joules:	Joules:	Joules:	Joules:

Medical Control: ☐ Direct ☐ C-MED Channel _____
MD# _____   Hospital _____
Hospital Notified Enroute: ☐ Yes   ☐ No
☐ C-MED ☐ Dispatcher
Other Response Units/Agencies: Police
#

E.M.S. TRAINING PROGRAM
PATIENT CARE REPORT FORM

© 1992 Kennedy Associates

Patient Name: Marybeth Herman
Address: 680 Washington St
Boston MA
DOB: 11/18/64   Tel. #: 555-8314
Next of Kin: Joanne Herman
Address: 10 Center Place
Boston MA
Relationship: Sister   Tel. #: 555-4011
Transported to: C.H.   Transport Priority: 2
Miles from: To:
☐ No Transport
REASON:

Trip #: 023   Date: 9/30/92
M.R.#:   Day: Wednesday
Dispatch To: For: Person struck by car
100 Riverbank Rd.
Dispatch Time: 0636   Arrival Time: 0641
To Hospital: At Hospital:
Location at Dispatch:
Billing Information (circle):
Medicare   Medicaid   BC/BS
Indust. Acc.   Self   Other
Subscriber:
Policy #:

Physical Exam

Eye Opening: ☒ Spontaneous   ☐ To Pain   ☐ To Voice   ☐ None

Verbal Response: ☒ Oriented   ☐ Confused   ☐ Inappropriate   ☐ Incomprehensible   ☐ None

Motor Response: ☒ Obedience   ☐ Purposeful   ☐ Withdrawal   ☐ Flexion   ☐ Extension   ☐ None

Skin Condition: ☒ Normal   ☐ Cool   ☐ Hot   ☐ Pale   ☐ Flushed   ☐ Cyanotic   ☐ Diaphoretic

Vital Signs

☐ Unable to Obtain   ☐ Not attempted
REASON:

Time	BP	Pulse	Resp. Rate/Effort
@ 0645	116/P	80 R	16

Allergies: NKA   ☐ None   ☐ Unknown

Current Medications: ∅   ☐ None   ☐ Unknown

Brought with Pt.? ☐ Yes   ☐ No

Suspected Diagnosis: ☐ Chronic   ☐ Acute
☐ Major Trauma ☐ Acute Medical ☐ Cardiac Arrest ☐ Shock
☒ Minor Trauma ☐ Minor Medical ☐ Cardiac Disorder ☐ ETOH
☐ Soft Tissue Injury ☐ Burns ☐ Ortho ☐ OD/Poison
☐ Neuro ☐ Seizure ☐ Psych ☐ OB/GYN ☐ Neonate

Emergency Care: ☐ CPR ☐ Extricate ☒ Back/Neck Immobilize
☐ Bleed Control ☐ Bandage ☐ Splint ☐ Heat/Cold Applied
☐ O2 Administration: _____ liters/minute via _____
Airway: ☐ Cleared ☐ Oral ☐ Nasal Size: _____ ☐ Suction
Intubate: ☐ Endotracheal ☐ Nasotracheal Size: _____
Assist Ventilation: Rate: _____ Method: _____
☐ ECG Monitor ☐ Rhythm Strip Attached
Transport Position: Supine

Chief Complaint/History/Changes in Patient Status

27 yo ♀ found sitting on sidewalk
c̄ C-spine collar on (Placed By
Fire Dept.) Pt c/c Head Pain p̄ MVA
c̄ Heavy exterior Damage ē Interior
intact. Winshield was spidered
on Passenger side. Pt. was
Passenger (restrained) unk speed
of vehicles prior to impact.
PMH: ∅ Rx: ∅ All: ∅
(PE) Pt A/Ox3 w/D Skin ē NAD
Post Head Presents Tenderness to
occipital Region of Head c̄ ⊖ Deformity
or signs of Inj. Anterior Presents
PEARL @ midpoint c̄ Numbness to R
cheek (some redness noted) ⊖ Deformity,
midline Trach BBS ≡ clear all fields
c̄ good volume, chest ↑↓ Symm.
ABD clear all Quads c̄ Pelvis
intact, upper/Lower Ext clear

Advanced Life Support

Time	Medication	Rate/Dose	Route
Pt C-spine immob to Hospital S.A			
		/	
		/	
		/	
		/	

Total Fluid Infused: _____ mls

DEFIB: Time:	Time:	Time:	Time:
Joules:	Joules:	Joules:	Joules:

Medical Control: ☐ Direct ☐ C-MED Channel _____
MD#: _____   Hospital _____
Hospital Notified Enroute: ☒ Yes ☐ No
☐ C-MED ☒ Dispatcher

Other Response Units/Agencies:
Police Dept.   Fire Dept.

Unit # A75   EMT/Paramedic Signatures: P. Bailey # 329   T. Johnson # 355   _____ # _____

E.M.S. TRAINING PROGRAM
PATIENT CARE REPORT FORM

© 1992 Kennedy Associates

Patient Name:	James Farrell	Trip #: 024		Date: 30 September 19
Address:	210 Woodland Ave	M.R.#:		Day: Wednesday
	Boston MA	Dispatch To:	For: Illness	
DOB: 10 July 1954	Tel. #: 555-6968	210 Woodland Ave		
Next of Kin: Deborah Farrell		Dispatch Time: 1:55	Arrival Time: 2:02	
Address: 210 Woodland Ave		To Hospital:	At Hospital:	
Boston MA		Location at Dispatch: Station 3		
Relationship: Wife	Tel. #: 555-6968	Billing Information (circle):		

Transported to: ___ Transport Priority: ___
Miles from: ___ To: ___

Billing Information (circle): Medicare   Medicaid   BC/BS
Indust. Acc.   Self   Other

❑ No Transport
REASON:

Subscriber: ___

Policy #: ___

Physical Exam

Eye Opening	☒ Spontaneous	❑ To Pain
	❑ To Voice	❑ None
Verbal Response	☒ Oriented	❑ Confused
	❑ Inappropriate	❑ Incomprehensible ❑ None
Motor Response	☒ Obedience	❑ Purposeful ❑ Withdrawal
	❑ Flexion	❑ Extension ❑ None
Skin Condition	❑ Normal ❑ Cool ☒ Hot ❑ Pale	
	❑ Flushed ❑ Cyanotic ❑ Diaphoretic	

Chief Complaint/History/Changes in Patient Status

38 y/o ♂ epigastric pain
(HPI) Pt states c ½° of epigastric
pain getting gradually worse.
Denies nausea, vomiting or Diarrhea
Denies Dyspnea Pain described as
sharp c varying intensity
(PMH) Environmental Allergies
(Meds) Seldane, psuedafed (NKDA)
(PE) cons A+Ox3, Skin warm & dry
EKG sinus @ 88 s ectopy. ⊖ JVD,
trachea midline. BS clear + = c Tidal
Volume. ABD soft Pain ↑ on
palpation of xyphoid area
(TX) transport s A

Vital Signs

❑ Unable to Obtain   ❑ Not attempted
REASON:

Time	BP	Pulse	Resp. Rate/Effort
2:05	116/78	88	16

Allergies: ☒ None   ❑ Unknown

Current Medications: Seldane   ❑ None   ❑ Unknown

Brought with Pt.?   ❑ Yes   ☒ No

Advanced Life Support

Time	/	Medication	/	Rate/Dose	/	Route
/		/		/		
/		/		/		
/		/		/		
/		/		/		
/		/		/		
/		/		/		
/		/		/		

Suspected Diagnosis: ❑ Chronic   ❑ Acute
❑ Major Trauma   ❑ Acute Medical   ❑ Cardiac Arrest   ❑ Shock
❑ Minor Trauma   ❑ Minor Medical   ❑ Cardiac Disorder   ❑ ETOH
❑ Soft Tissue Injury   ❑ Burns   ❑ Ortho   ❑ OD/Poison
❑ Neuro   ❑ Seizure   ❑ Psych   ❑ OB/GYN   ❑ Neonate

Total Fluid Infused: ___ mls

Emergency Care: ❑ CPR   ❑ Extricate   ❑ Back/Neck Immobilize
❑ Bleed Control   ❑ Bandage   ❑ Splint   ❑ Heat/Cold Applied
❑ O₂ Administration: ___ liters/minute via ___
Airway: ❑ Cleared   ❑ Oral   ❑ Nasal Size: ___   ❑ Suction
Intubate: ❑ Endotracheal   ❑ Nasotracheal Size: ___
Assist Ventilation: Rate: ___   Method: ___
☒ ECG Monitor   ❑ Rhythm Strip Attached
Transport Position: Seated c belts

DEFIB: Time: ___ Time: ___ Time: ___ Time: ___
Joules: ___ Joules: ___ Joules: ___ Joules: ___
Medical Control: ❑ Direct   ❑ C-MED Channel ___
MD# ___ Hospital ___
Hospital Notified Enroute: ❑ Yes   ❑ No
❑ C-MED   ❑ Dispatcher

Other Response Units/Agencies: ___

Unit # 16   EMT/Paramedic Signatures: J. Louden   # 178   K. Devine   # 182   ___ #

E.M.S. TRAINING PROGRAM
PATIENT CARE REPORT FORM

© 1992 Kennedy Associates

Patient Name: Stephanie Draftman	Trip #: 025 Date: 9/30/92
Address: 146 Richmore Road Randolph MA	M.R.#: 015 60 20 Day: Wed.
DOB: 2/18/23 Tel. #: 555-9681	Dispatch To: 146 Richmore rd. For: Illness
Next of Kin: Jonathan Draftman	Dispatch Time: 0808 Arrival Time: 0816
Address: Same	To Hospital: 0828 At Hospital: 0840
	Location at Dispatch: Quarters

Relationship: Husband   Tel. #: Same
Transported to: Community Hosp   Transport Priority: 2
Miles from: 1628.5   To 1649.2
☐ No Transport
REASON:

Billing Information (circle): **(Medicare)**   Medicaid   BC/BS
   Indust. Acc.   Self   Other
Subscriber: Jonathan Draftman
Policy #: 0302050 61 B

Physical Exam

Eye Opening	☒ Spontaneous	☐ To Pain
	☐ To Voice	☐ None
Verbal Response	☒ Oriented	☐ Confused
	☐ Inappropriate	☐ Incomprehensible ☐ None
Motor Response	☒ Obedience	☐ Purposeful ☐ Withdrawal
	☐ Flexion	☐ Extension ☐ None
Skin Condition	☐ Normal ☐ Cool ☒ Hot ☐ Pale	
	☐ Flushed ☐ Cyanotic ☒ Diaphoretic	

Vital Signs

☐ Unable to Obtain   ☐ Not attempted
REASON:

Time	BP	Pulse	Resp. Rate/Effort
0821	138/60	96 R	24 NL

Allergies: NKDA

Current Medications: See ®

☒ None ☐ Unknown
☐ None ☐ Unknown

Brought with Pt.? ☐ Yes ☐ No

Suspected Diagnosis: ☐ Chronic ☐ Acute
☐ Major Trauma ☐ Acute Medical ☐ Cardiac Arrest ☐ Shock
☐ Minor Trauma ☐ Minor Medical ☐ Cardiac Disorder ☐ ETOH
☐ Soft Tissue Injury ☐ Burns ☐ Ortho ☐ OD/Poison
☐ Neuro ☐ Seizure ☐ Psych ☐ OB/GYN ☐ Neonate

Chief Complaint/History/Changes in Patient Status

69 yo ♀ c/o Headache
Pt. states headache centered in frontal region x 12 hr. Pt denies any Hx of same states she has had minor headaches of the same type c̄ a asthma attack. States she had some symptoms of her asthma ~ 6 HR which was relieved by her ventolin nebulizer. Also c/o nausea c̄ vomiting x 2 days
⊖ SOB, dizziness

PE - CA Ox3. Skin hot diaphoretic +1 lungs - clear Eq. Bilat. c̄ ⊕ TV PERL ⊖ evidence of Resp. distress Remainder of exam unremarkable

PMH - Asthma, HTN
MED - Vent. Nebulizer Q 4 Hr Vasotec, Tavist, Cephlaxin Prednisone (DC'ed x 2 wk)
NKDA

Advanced Life Support

Time	/ Medication	/ Rate/Dose	/ Route
Rx — Transport/	3 A	/	
/		/	/
/		/	/
/		/	/
/		/	/
/		/	/
/		/	/

Total Fluid Infused: _____ mls

Emergency Care: ☐ CPR ☐ Extricate ☐ Back/Neck Immobilize
☐ Bleed Control ☐ Bandage ☐ Splint ☐ Heat/Cold Applied
☐ O₂ Administration: _____ liters/minute via _____
Airway: ☐ Cleared ☐ Oral ☐ Nasal Size: _____ ☐ Suction
Intubate: ☐ Endotracheal ☐ Nasotracheal Size: _____
Assist Ventilation: Rate: _____ Method: _____
☐ ECG Monitor ☐ Rhythm Strip Attached
Transport Position: Semi-fowlers

DEFIB:	Time:	Time:	Time:	Time:
	Joules:	Joules:	Joules:	Joules:

Medical Control: ☐ Direct ☐ C-MED Channel _____
MD#_____ Hospital _____
Hospital Notified Enroute: ☐ Yes ☐ No
☐ C-MED ☐ Dispatcher

Other Response Units/Agencies:

Unit # A 37
EMT/Paramedic Signatures:
_____   # _____   # _____

E.M.S. TRAINING PROGRAM
PATIENT CARE REPORT FORM

© 1992 Kennedy Associates

Patient Name: Thomas Casey	Trip #: 026 Date: 9/30/92
Address: 5 Brookfield Lane	M.R.#: Day: Wed.
Weston MA	Dispatch To: For: person fell
DOB: 10/28/63 Tel. #: 555-4262	5 Brookfield Lane
Next of Kin: Mary Casey	Dispatch Time: 2056 Arrival Time: 2101
Address: Same	To Hospital: At Hospital:
	Location at Dispatch:
Relationship: Sister Tel. #: Same	Billing Information (circle):
Transported to: T.G.H. Transport Priority: 3	Medicare Medicaid (BC/BS)
Miles from: To:	Indust. Acc. Self Other
❏ No Transport	Subscriber: Thomas Casey
REASON:	
	Policy #: 060 974632

Physical Exam

Eye Opening	☒ Spontaneous ❏ To Pain
	❏ To Voice ❏ None
Verbal Response	☒ Oriented ❏ Confused
	❏ Inappropriate ❏ Incomprehensible ❏ None
Motor Response	☒ Obedience ❏ Purposeful ❏ Withdrawal
	❏ Flexion ❏ Extension ❏ None
Skin Condition	☒ Normal ❏ Cool ❏ Hot ❏ Pale
	❏ Flushed ❏ Cyanotic ❏ Diaphoretic

Vital Signs

❏ Unable to Obtain   ❏ Not attempted

REASON:

Time	BP	Pulse	Resp. Rate/Effort
2108	150/84	96R	36

Allergies:	❏ None
	☒ Unknown
Current Medications:	❏ None
	☒ Unknown

Brought with Pt.?   ❏ Yes   ❏ No

Suspected Diagnosis: ❏ Chronic   ❏ Acute

❏ Major Trauma ❏ Acute Medical ❏ Cardiac Arrest ❏ Shock
❏ Minor Trauma ❏ Minor Medical ❏ Cardiac Disorder ❏ ETOH
☒ Soft Tissue Injury ❏ Burns ❏ Ortho ❏ OD/Poison
❏ Neuro ❏ Seizure ❏ Psych ❏ OB/GYN ❏ Neonate

Emergency Care: ❏ CPR ❏ Extricate ❏ Back/Neck Immobilize
❏ Bleed Control ❏ Bandage ☒ Splint ❏ Heat/Cold Applied
❏ O₂ Administration: _____ liters/minute via _____
Airway: ❏ Cleared ☒ Oral ❏ Nasal Size: _____ ❏ Suction
Intubate: ❏ Endotracheal ❏ Nasotracheal Size: _____
Assist Ventilation: Rate: _____ Method: _____
❏ ECG Monitor ❏ Rhythm Strip Attached
Transport Position: Supine

Unit # A78   EMT/Paramedic Signatures: J.G. #_____   M.H. #_____   #_____

Chief Complaint/History/Changes in Patient Status

28yo ♂ found supine on floor of bathroom after folding table legs gave out + struck his Ⓡ shin c/o Ø feeling in arms or legs secondary c/o tingeling in arms. Pt. Hyperventilat PE: CA+O, skin warm and dry pup =/react @ 4mm Head + neck ⊖ chest sym. c=/Bilat breath sounds ABD + Pelvis ⊖ ⊕ motor resp. moving arms + legs during exam + during B/P

PMH: unkn   meds: unkn
Allg: unkn

Pt transported to hospital s̄ Δ or incident

Advanced Life Support

Time	/	Medication	/	Rate/Dose	/	Route
	/		/		/	
	/		/		/	
	/		/		/	
	/		/		/	
	/		/		/	
	/		/		/	

Total Fluid Infused: _____ mls

DEFIB: Time:	Time:	Time:	Time:
Joules:	Joules:	Joules:	Joules:

Medical Control: ❏ Direct ❏ C-MED Channel _____
MD#_____   Hospital _____
Hospital Notified Enroute: ❏ Yes ☒ No
❏ C-MED ❏ Dispatcher

Other Response Units/Agencies:

E.M.S. TRAINING PROGRAM
PATIENT CARE REPORT FORM

© 1992 Kennedy Associates

Patient Name: Jason Bliss	Trip #: 027 — Date: 9/30/92
Address: 400 Main St.	M.R.#: — Day: Wed.
Hartford Conn.	Dispatch To: 20 Lincoln Ave — For: Illness
DOB: 12-20-33 Tel. #: 555-2967	
Next of Kin:	Dispatch Time: — Arrival Time:
Address:	To Hospital: — At Hospital:
	Location at Dispatch:
Relationship: — Tel. #:	Billing Information (circle):
Transported to: T.G.H. — Transport Priority:	Medicare Medicaid BC/BS
Miles from: — To:	Indust. Acc. (Self) Other
❑ No Transport	Subscriber:
REASON:	
	Policy #:

Physical Exam

Eye Opening	☑ Spontaneous ❑ To Pain	
	❑ To Voice ❑ None	
Verbal Response	❑ Oriented ❑ Confused	
	☑ Inappropriate ❑ Incomprehensible ❑ None	
Motor Response	☑ Obedience ❑ Purposeful ❑ Withdrawal	
	❑ Flexion ❑ Extension ❑ None	
Skin Condition	☑ Normal ❑ Cool ❑ Hot ❑ Pale	
	❑ Flushed ❑ Cyanotic ❑ Diaphoretic	

Vital Signs

❑ Unable to Obtain   ❑ Not attempted
REASON: Uncooperative

Time	BP	Pulse	Resp. Rate/Effort

Chief Complaint/History/Changes in Patient Status

Altered Mental Status
58 yo MALE c̄ history manic
depression Presented seated
in Police car Pt consc Alert x 3,
Pt sts compliance with meds,
Pt's associate sts ∅ compliance
x 1 week
Pt sts he wants to sign in to
McLean Hospital For Evaluation.
Pt was transported Seated
status unchanging enroute
transport uneventful.
Pt was met by security at Hospital

Allergies: Unknown — ❑ None   ☒ Unknown

Current Medications: non-compliant — ❑ None   ❑ Unknown

PMH: Manic Depression

Brought with Pt.?   ❑ Yes   ❑ No

Advanced Life Support

Time	Medication	Rate/Dose	Route
MEDS	Lithium		
	Prozac		
Allerg	unknown		

Total Fluid Infused: _____ mls

Suspected Diagnosis: ❑ Chronic   ❑ Acute
❑ Major Trauma   ❑ Acute Medical   ❑ Cardiac Arrest   ❑ Shock
❑ Minor Trauma   ❑ Minor Medical   ❑ Cardiac Disorder   ❑ ETOH
❑ Soft Tissue Injury   ❑ Burns   ❑ Ortho   ❑ OD/Poison
❑ Neuro   ❑ Seizure   ❑ Psych   ❑ OB/GYN   ❑ Neonate

DEFIB:	Time:	Time:	Time:	Time:
	Joules:	Joules:	Joules:	Joules:

Emergency Care: ❑ CPR   ❑ Extricate   ❑ Back/Neck Immobilize
❑ Bleed Control   ❑ Bandage   ❑ Splint   ❑ Heat/Cold Applied
❑ O₂ Administration: _____ liters/minute via _____
Airway: ❑ Cleared   ❑ Oral   ❑ Nasal Size: _____   ❑ Suction
Intubate: ❑ Endotracheal   ❑ Nasotracheal Size: _____
Assist Ventilation: Rate: _____   Method: _____
❑ ECG Monitor   ❑ Rhythm Strip Attached
Transport Position: Seated

Medical Control: ❑ Direct   ❑ C-MED Channel _____
MD# _____   Hospital _____
Hospital Notified Enroute: ❑ Yes   ☑ No
❑ C-MED   ❑ Dispatcher

Other Response Units/Agencies:
Police

Unit # A8   EMT/Paramedic Signatures:
Phyllis Lush #_____   Tim Martin #_____   #_____

E.M.S. TRAINING PROGRAM
PATIENT CARE REPORT FORM

© 1992 Kennedy Associates

Patient Name: George Blank
Address: 88 Columbia Ave
Boston Ma
DOB: 11-10-50   Tel. #: 555-2632
Next of Kin: Joe Johnson
Address: S/A

Relationship: Friend   Tel. #: Some
Transported to: T.G.H   Transport Priority: 3
Miles from: 10506.2   To: 10521.6
❏ No Transport
REASON:

Trip #: 028   Date: Sept. 30 1992
M.R.#:   Day: Wed
Dispatch To: For: Psychiatric Emergency
Tom's Place
Dispatch Time: Arrival Time:
To Hospital: At Hospital:
Location at Dispatch:
Billing Information (circle):
          Medicare   Medicaid   BC/BS
          Indust. Acc.   Self   Other
Subscriber:

Policy #:

Physical Exam

Eye Opening: ☒ Spontaneous   ❏ To Pain   ❏ To Voice   ❏ None
Verbal Response: ☒ Oriented   ❏ Confused   ❏ Inappropriate   ❏ Incomprehensible   ❏ None
Motor Response: ☒ Obedience   ❏ Purposeful   ❏ Withdrawal   ❏ Flexion   ❏ Extension   ❏ None
Skin Condition: ☒ Normal   ❏ Cool   ❏ Hot   ❏ Pale   ❏ Flushed   ❏ Cyanotic   ❏ Diaphoretic

Vital Signs

❏ Unable to Obtain   ❏ Not attempted
REASON:

Time	BP	Pulse	Resp. Rate/Effort
	170/94	80	18

Allergies: UNK   ❏ None   ❏ Unknown

Current Medications: ⟶   ❏ None   ❏ Unknown

Brought with Pt.?   ❏ Yes   ☒ No

Chief Complaint/History/Changes in Patient Status

42 yo ♂ Homicidal
Pt Found sitting in Yaway House
of For Psych. Disorders & substance
Abuse. 6 mo program c̄ 2 day left
became aggitated in a group
session and went to chief of Staff
Homicidal c̄ A specific IDEATION of
killing 2 of the group participants
Now in control & "cooling out..."
Presented a Threat during transp
PMH: Depression, Angina, HTSN
MEDS: PROZAC, NIFEDIPINE,
IBUPROFEN, BALLOFEN
CYPRONE PADINE
NKDA

Suspected Diagnosis: ☒ Chronic   ☒ Acute
❏ Major Trauma   ❏ Acute Medical   ❏ Cardiac Arrest   ❏ Shock
❏ Minor Trauma   ❏ Minor Medical   ❏ Cardiac Disorder   ❏ ETOH
❏ Soft Tissue Injury   ❏ Burns   ❏ Ortho   ❏ OD/Poison
❏ Neuro   ❏ Seizure   ☒ Psych   ❏ OB/GYN   ❏ Neonate

Advanced Life Support

Time	/	Medication	/	Rate/Dose	/	Route
	/		/		/	
	/		/		/	
	/		/		/	
	/		/		/	
	/		/		/	
	/		/		/	

Total Fluid Infused: mls

Emergency Care: ❏ CPR   ❏ Extricate   ❏ Back/Neck Immobilize
❏ Bleed Control   ❏ Bandage   ❏ Splint   ❏ Heat/Cold Applied
❏ O₂ Administration: _____ liters/minute via _____
Airway: ❏ Cleared   ❏ Oral   ❏ Nasal   Size: _____   ❏ Suction
Intubate: ❏ Endotracheal   ❏ Nasotracheal   Size: _____
Assist Ventilation: Rate: _____   Method: _____
❏ ECG Monitor   ❏ Rhythm Strip Attached
Transport Position: Sitting

DEFIB: Time: Time: Time: Time:
          Joules: Joules: Joules: Joules:
Medical Control: ❏ Direct   ❏ C-MED   Channel _____
MD#_____   Hospital _____
Hospital Notified Enroute: ❏ Yes   ❏ No
                    ❏ C-MED   ❏ Dispatcher
Other Response Units/Agencies: Police

Unit # A32
EMT/Paramedic Signatures: Bill Monroe   #_____   _____ #_____   _____ #_____

E.M.S. TRAINING PROGRAM
PATIENT CARE REPORT FORM

© 1992 Kennedy Associates

Patient Name: Ralph Martins	Trip #: 029 Date: 9/30/92
Address: Unknown	M.R.#: Day: Wednesday
	Dispatch To: For: Assault/
DOB: Unknown Tel. #:	50 King ST
Next of Kin:	Dispatch Time: 1828 Arrival Time: 1836
Address:	To Hospital: 1845 At Hospital: 1855
	Location at Dispatch: Quarters
Relationship: Tel. #:	Billing Information (circle):
Transported to: Trauma Gen. Hos, Transport Priority: 3	Medicare Medicaid BC/BS
Miles from: To:	Indust. Acc. Self Other
☐ No Transport	Subscriber:
REASON:	
	Policy #:

Physical Exam

Eye Opening	☒ Spontaneous ☐ To Pain	
	☐ To Voice ☐ None	
Verbal Response	☐ Oriented ☐ Confused	
	☐ Inappropriate ☐ Incomprehensible ☐ None	
Motor Response	☐ Obedience ☒ Purposeful ☐ Withdrawal	
	☐ Flexion ☐ Extension ☐ None	
Skin Condition	☒ Normal ☐ Cool ☐ Hot ☐ Pale	
	☐ Flushed ☐ Cyanotic ☐ Diaphoretic	

Vital Signs

☐ Unable to Obtain   ☐ Not attempted

REASON:

Time	BP	Pulse	Resp. Rate/Effort
1842	140/78	80	14

Allergies: ☐ None ☒ Unknown

Current Medications: ☐ None ☒ Unknown

Brought with Pt.?   ☐ Yes   ☐ No

Suspected Diagnosis: ☐ Chronic   ☐ Acute
☐ Major Trauma ☐ Acute Medical ☐ Cardiac Arrest ☐ Shock
☐ Minor Trauma ☐ Minor Medical ☐ Cardiac Disorder ☐ ETOH
☒ Soft Tissue Injury ☐ Burns ☒ Ortho? ☐ OD/Poison
☐ Neuro ☐ Seizure ☐ Psych ☐ OB/GYN ☐ Neonate

Chief Complaint/History/Changes in Patient Status

Assault victim — Nose bleed
35 YO W♂ who was assaulted by a
few men (3 or 4) Punching and Kicking
Pt according to witnesses.
Pt found Lying on ® side appears
ETOH opens eyes on command has
some blood on his nose Maybe some
deformity to nose but appears old.
Pt becomes verbally abusive when
asked any questions at all. Refused
to give any clue to incident or nature
of any injury. Becomes combative
when touched. Does have Purposeful
movement — PEARL at 5mm Skin warm
and dry chest and abdomen unremarkable
on exam and that is all pt. would
allow for P/E
PmH = unk
meds = unk
Allerg = unk

Advanced Life Support

Time	/	Medication	/	Rate/Dose	/	Route
	/		/		/	
	/		/		/	
	/		/		/	
	/		/		/	
	/		/		/	
	/		/		/	

Total Fluid Infused: mls

Emergency Care: ☐ CPR ☐ Extricate ☒ Back/Neck Immobilize
☐ Bleed Control ☐ Bandage ☐ Splint ☐ Heat/Cold Applied
☐ O₂ Administration: _____ liters/minute via _____
Airway: ☐ Cleared ☐ Oral ☐ Nasal Size: _____ ☐ Suction
Intubate: ☐ Endotracheal ☐ Nasotracheal Size: _____
Assist Ventilation: Rate: _____ Method: _____
☐ ECG Monitor ☐ Rhythm Strip Attached
Transport Position: Supine

DEFIB: Time: Time: Time: Time:
Joules: Joules: Joules: Joules:

Medical Control: ☐ Direct ☐ C-MED Channel _____
MD#_____   Hospital _____
Hospital Notified Enroute: ☐ Yes   ☐ No
☐ C-MED ☐ Dispatcher

Other Response Units/Agencies:

Unit # A16   EMT/Paramedic Signatures: Patrick Jewell #322   Sue Patton #336   #_____

E.M.S. TRAINING PROGRAM
PATIENT CARE REPORT FORM

© 1992 Kennedy Associat[es]

Patient Name: Maureen Perry	Trip #: 030 Date: Sept. 30 '92
Address: 25 mansfield Road	M.R.#: Day: Wed.
Boston MA	Dispatch To: For: assault
DOB: 10-08-66 Tel. #: 555-3711	midtown station
Next of Kin:	Dispatch Time: 1800 Arrival Time: 1805
Address:	To Hospital: At Hospital:
	Location at Dispatch: station 1
Relationship: Tel. #:	Billing Information (circle):
Transported to: C.H. Transport Priority:	Medicare Medicaid BC/BS
Miles from: To:	Indust. Acc. Self Other
❏ No Transport	Subscriber:
REASON:	
	Policy #:

Physical Exam

Eye Opening: ☒ Spontaneous ❏ To Pain ❏ To Voice ❏ None

Verbal Response: ☒ Oriented ❏ Confused ❏ Inappropriate ❏ Incomprehensible ❏ None

Motor Response: ☒ Obedience ❏ Purposeful ❏ Withdrawal ❏ Flexion ❏ Extension ❏ None

Skin Condition: ☒ Normal ❏ Cool ❏ Hot ❏ Pale ❏ Flushed ❏ Cyanotic ❏ Diaphoretic

Vital Signs

❏ Unable to Obtain   ❏ Not attempted
REASON:

Time	BP	Pulse	Resp. Rate/Effort
1809	100/70	88	20

Allergies: NKDA   ☒ None ❏ Unknown

Current Medications: ☒ None ❏ Unknown

Brought with Pt.? ❏ Yes ❏ No

Suspected Diagnosis: ❏ Chronic ❏ Acute
❏ Major Trauma ❏ Acute Medical ❏ Cardiac Arrest ❏ Shock
❏ Minor Trauma ☒ Minor Medical ❏ Cardiac Disorder ❏ ETOH
❏ Soft Tissue Injury ❏ Burns ❏ Ortho ❏ OD/Poison
❏ Neuro ❏ Seizure ❏ Psych ❏ OB/GYN ❏ Neonate

Emergency Care: ❏ CPR ❏ Extricate ❏ Back/Neck Immobilize
❏ Bleed Control ❏ Bandage ❏ Splint ❏ Heat/Cold Applied
❏ O₂ Administration: _____ liters/minute via _____
Airway: ❏ Cleared ❏ Oral ❏ Nasal Size: _____ ❏ Suction
Intubate: ❏ Endotracheal ❏ Nasotracheal Size: _____
Assist Ventilation: Rate: _____ Method: _____
❏ ECG Monitor ❏ Rhythm Strip Attached
Transport Position: Seated

Unit # A29   EMT/Paramedic Signatures:
#_____ #_____ #_____

Chief Complaint/History/Changes in Patient Status

25 yo ♀ found @ above w/ Transi[t]
Police who states was Sexually
assaulted by individual w/assaila[nt]
dragging Pt over cement attempt[ing]
to strangle victim via hands. Pt
Stating assault took place between 1600-1730. Pt found slig[ht]-
ly anxious. w/moderate size abr[as]-
ion to Ⓡ post. shoulder area.
Pt states she was not choked
into unconsciousness. Further
unrem.
PMH: ∅
Med: ∅
Aller: ∅
unknown last tetanus w/∅
Δ's enroute to hosp

Advanced Life Support

Time	/	Medication	/	Rate/Dose	/	Route
	/		/		/	
	/		/		/	
	/		/		/	
	/		/		/	
	/		/		/	
	/		/		/	
	/		/		/	

Total Fluid Infused: _____ mls

DEFIB: Time: Time: Time: Time:
Joules: Joules: Joules: Joules:

Medical Control: ❏ Direct ❏ C-MED Channel _____
MD#_____ Hospital _____
Hospital Notified Enroute: ❏ Yes ❏ No
❏ C-MED ❏ Dispatcher

Other Response Units/Agencies:
Police (Transit)

Notes

E.M.S. TRAINING PROGRAM
PATIENT CARE REPORT FORM

© 1992 Kennedy Associates

Patient Name: Daniel Perkins	Trip #: 031 Date: Sept. 30 '92
Address: 49 Case St.	M.R.#: Day: Wed.
Boston MA	Dispatch To: For: Illness ? Diabet
DOB: Dec 2 '30 Tel. #: 555-2469	100 Wash. St. - BiRightmachines Co.
Next of Kin: Frances	Dispatch Time: 1042 Arrival Time: 1045
Address: Same	To Hospital: 1107 At Hospital: 1111
	Location at Dispatch: Station 4

Relationship: wife   Tel. #: Same
Transported to: Community Hosp.   Transport Priority: 3
Miles from: To:
❏ No Transport
REASON:

Billing Information (circle):
Medicare   Medicaid   (BC/BS)
Indust. Acc.   Self   Other

Subscriber: Patient
(Group Plan - employer (see above)
Policy #:

Physical Exam

Eye Opening	☒ Spontaneous ❏ To Pain ❏ To Voice ❏ None
Verbal Response	❏ Oriented ❏ Confused ❏ Inappropriate ☒ Incomprehensible ❏ None
Motor Response	❏ Obedience ❏ Purposeful ❏ Withdrawal ❏ Flexion ❏ Extension ☒ None
Skin Condition	❏ Normal ❏ Cool ❏ Hot ☒ Pale ❏ Flushed ❏ Cyanotic ☒ Diaphoretic

Chief Complaint/History/Changes in Patient Status

AMS
62 y/o w ♂ coworkers called - ↑ AMS
PE ❍ verbal respones understood, ↓ tdia
pale, IV D5W KVO, Bloods drawn
40 mg/dl 18 1/4 C 100mg Thiamine
1 amp D50 pt mentation ↑ A/0x2
To name & place 2nd amp D50
- skin Drier - A/0x3.

Vital Signs

❏ Unable to Obtain   ❏ Not attempted
REASON:

Time	BP	Pulse	Resp. Rate/Effort
1105	142/90	50 ⇒	20
		30	
		50	

BP 142/90 EKG 1° AVB @ 50 Invert
T II III, mCl, mCl₆ HR ↓ 30, S/P D50
EKG T 1° AVB @ SB T waves invert
still.   15l nonreb O₂ /Switched from
4l nasal initially placed on)
PMH recent Dx Diab & HTN
MEDS Insulin & antihypertensive
unk Alleg

Allergies: ❏ None
UNK   ❏ Unknown

Rx Eval O₂ IV monitor Tport C ↑ MS
& pt Verbalizing A/0x3

Current Medications: ❏ None
Insulin & anti HTN meds   ❏ Unknown

Advanced Life Support

Time	Medication	Rate/Dose	Route
1105	D5W	KVO	18 1/4" ②
1105	thiamine	100mg	IV WMISS
1106	D50	1 amp	IV
1110	D50	1 amp	IV
/	/	/	
/	/	/	
/	/	/	
/	/	/	

Brought with Pt.? ❏ Yes ❏ No

Suspected Diagnosis: ❏ Chronic ❏ Acute
❏ Major Trauma ❏ Acute Medical ❏ Cardiac Arrest ❏ Shock
❏ Minor Trauma ❏ Minor Medical ❏ Cardiac Disorder ❏ ETOH
❏ Soft Tissue Injury ❏ Burns ❏ Ortho ❏ OD/Poison
❏ Neuro ❏ Seizure ❏ Psych ❏ OB/GYN ❏ Neonate

Total Fluid Infused: mls

Emergency Care: ❏ CPR ❏ Extricate ❏ Back/Neck Immobilize
❏ Bleed Control ❏ Bandage ❏ Splint ❏ Heat/Cold Applied
☒ O₂ Administration: 4l-15l liters/minute via Nasal→nonreb
Airway: ❏ Cleared ❏ Oral ❏ Nasal Size: _____ ❏ Suction
Intubate: ❏ Endotracheal ❏ Nasotracheal Size: _____
Assist Ventilation: Rate: _____ Method: _____
❏ ECG Monitor ❏ Rhythm Strip Attached
Transport Position: Semi-fowler

DEFIB:	Time:	Time:	Time:	Time:
	Joules:	Joules:	Joules:	Joules:

Medical Control: ❏ Direct ❏ C-MED Channel _____
MD# 62   Hospital _____
Hospital Notified Enroute: ❏ Yes ❏ No
    ❏ C-MED ❏ Dispatcher

Other Response Units/Agencies:

Unit # P4   EMT/Paramedic Signatures:
    J. Mayns   # 165   Crisp   # 168   #

Trip # 031

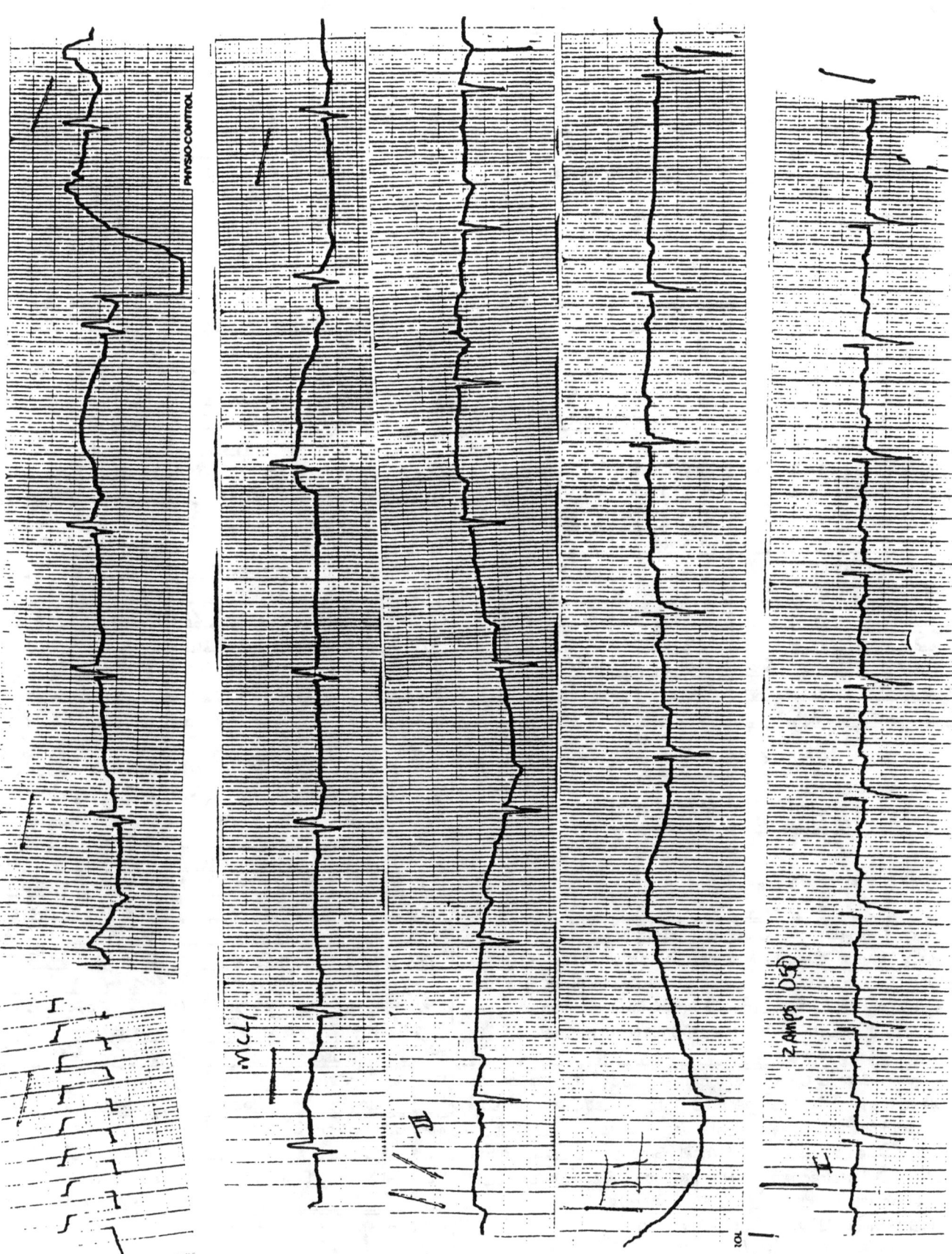

E.M.S. TRAINING PROGRAM
PATIENT CARE REPORT FORM

© 1992 Kennedy Associate

Patient Name: *Lawrence Norton*	Trip #: **032** Date: *Sept. 30 '92*
Address: *135 Chestnut St*	M.R.#: Day: *Wed.*
Medway MA	Dispatch To: For:
DOB: *4-8-32* Tel. #: *555-6234*	*Airport* *Gate 50*
Next of Kin: *Christine*	Dispatch Time: **820** Arrival Time: **826**
Address: *S/a*	To Hospital: **858** At Hospital: **905**
	Location at Dispatch:
Relationship: *Wife* Tel. #: *Same*	Billing Information (circle):
Transported to: *TGH* Transport Priority:	Medicare Medicaid BC/BS
Miles from: *604.8* To: *612.4* *1*	Indust. Acc. Self (Other)
☐ No Transport	*HMO*
REASON:	Subscriber:
	Policy #:

Physical Exam / Chief Complaint/History/Changes in Patient Status

Chief Complaint/History/Changes in Patient Status

Resp. Diff

60 y/o w ♂ at the airport flying out, c/o CP & SOB Took 2 NTG ØA (0.3mg) on arrive Pt. Removed from plane on O2 Pē cons, antietous. Ø verbal use of accessory muscles to breath RR 36 pt resp. status very poor Rales bases to ↑ apex bilat 4+ Diap, pale, unk CP pt not able to indicat Rest of exam unremarkable (VS) 210/P HR ST 130 c̄ frequent unifocal PVCs RR 34 (TX) Eval O2 15l non reb, monitor access poor ® hand line ① 20g 14, line ② 18s 14 → SL NTGs 0.4mg (Diff pt not wanting to open mouth) 2mg MSO4 BP 190/120 EKG ØA, 40mg Lasix 2nd 2mg MSO4 BP 190/P 2nd 40mg Lasix 2 SL NTG spray 0.4mg BP 160/P 2nd 4mg MSO4 — pt RR still 34 pt tire #6 Nasal ETT in ® nare (Rales) Good Brea Sounds c̄ Ambo, arrive at Hospital

Physical Exam:

Eye Opening	☒ Spontaneous ☐ To Pain	
	☐ To Voice ☐ None	
Verbal Response	☐ Oriented ☐ Confused	
	☐ Inappropriate ☐ Incomprehensible ☒ None	
Motor Response	☒ Obedience ☐ Purposeful ☐ Withdrawal	
	☒ Flexion ☐ Extension ☐ None	
Skin Condition	☐ Normal ☐ Cool ☐ Hot ☒ Pale *4+*	
	☐ Flushed ☐ Cyanotic ☒ Diaphoretic	

Vital Signs

☐ Unable to Obtain   ☐ Not attempted
REASON:

Time	BP	Pulse	Resp. Rate/Effort
851	210/P	130 irr	34
857	190/120	130 irr	34
904	160/P	130 irr	34

Allergies: *UNK*   ☐ None
                              ☐ Unknown

Current Medications: ☐ None
Lasix NTG   ☐ Unknown
Diabeta slow Po

Brought with Pt.? ☐ Yes ☐ No

Suspected Diagnosis: ☐ Chronic ☒ Acute
☐ Major Trauma ☒ Acute Medical ☐ Cardiac Arrest ☐ Shock
☐ Minor Trauma ☐ Minor Medical ☐ Cardiac Disorder ☐ ETOH
☐ Soft Tissue Injury ☐ Burns ☐ Ortho ☐ OD/Poison
☐ Neuro ☐ Seizure ☐ Psych ☐ OB/GYN ☐ Neonate

Advanced Life Support

Time	/	Medication	/	Rate/Dose	/	Route
0854	/	NTG	/	0.4mg	/	SL
0856	/	MSO4	/	2mg	/	IV
0857	/	Lasix	/	40mg	/	IV
0859	/	MSO4	/	2mg	/	IV
0901	/	Lasix	/	40mg	/	IV
0903/0904	/	NTG/NTG	/	0.4mg/0.4mg	/	IV IV
0904	/	MSO4	/	4mg	/	IV

Total Fluid Infused: ____ mls 2 D5W KVO ® Head 2 ® arm 18

Emergency Care:
☐ CPR ☐ Extricate ☐ Back/Neck Immobilize
☐ Bleed Control ☐ Bandage ☐ Splint ☐ Heat/Cold Applied
☒ O2 Administration: *15* liters/minute via *Nasal ET non reb*
Airway: ☐ Cleared ☐ Oral ☐ Nasal Size: ____ ☐ Suction
Intubate: ☐ Endotracheal ☒ Nasotracheal Size: *6*
Assist Ventilation: Rate: ____ Method: ____
☒ ECG Monitor ☐ Rhythm Strip Attached
Transport Position: *Fowler*

DEFIB: Time: ____ Time: ____ Time: ____ Time: ____
        Joules: ____ Joules: ____ Joules: ____ Joules: ____
Medical Control: ☐ Direct ☐ C-MED Channel ____
MD# **39**   Hospital ____
Hospital Notified Enroute: ☐ Yes ☐ No
                           ☐ C-MED ☐ Dispatcher
Other Response Units/Agencies:

Unit # *P10*   EMT/Paramedic Signatures: *Miley Barrett* # *182*   *Thomas Murry* # *190*   #

Trip #032

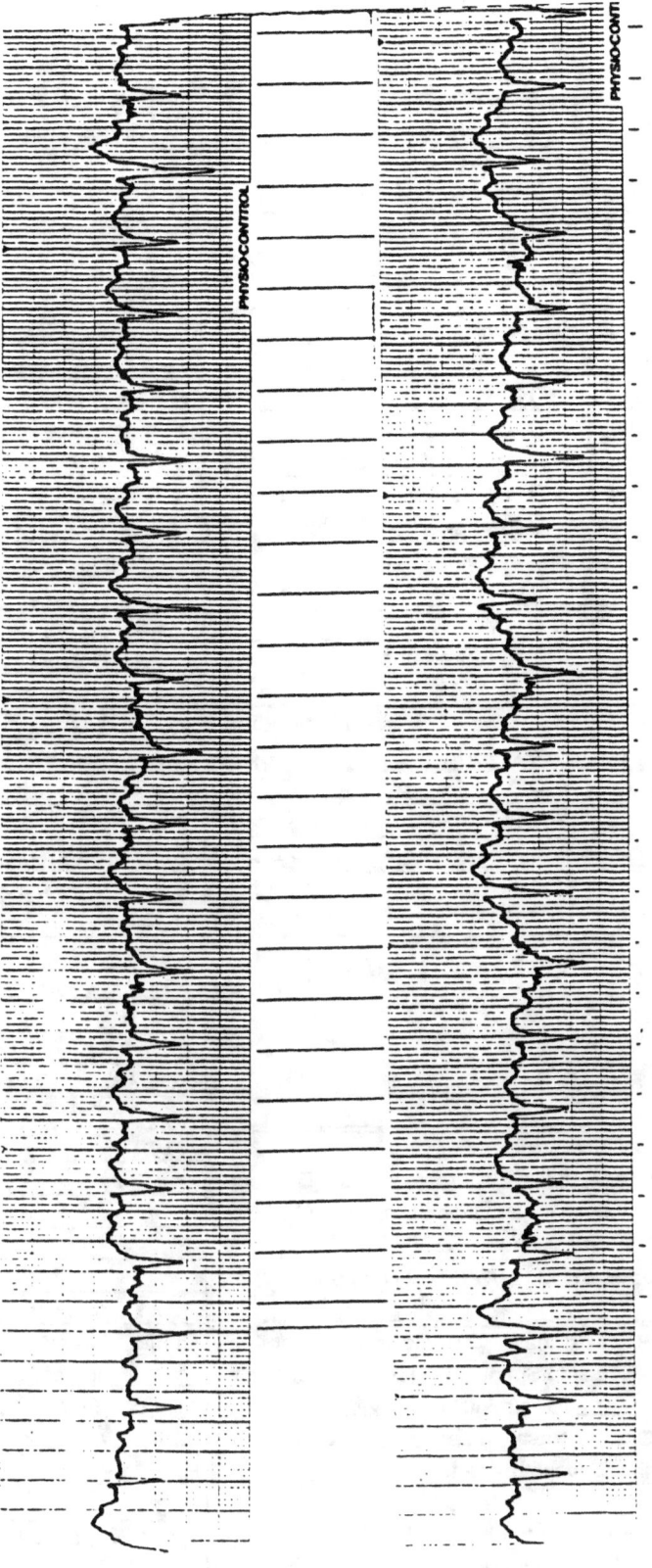

E.M.S. TRAINING PROGRAM
PATIENT CARE REPORT FORM

© 1992 Kennedy Associates

Patient Name: David Mahan	Trip #: 033 Date: 9-30-92
Address: 98 memorial Rd	M.R.#: Day: Wed.
Boston MA	Dispatch To: For: Injury
DOB: 11-19-42 Tel. #: 555-1404	Joe's Express - 40 Dalton Way
Next of Kin: Jennifer	Dispatch Time 0753 Arrival Time: 0801
Address: Same	To Hospital: 0823 At Hospital: 0832

Location at Dispatch:

Relationship: Wife   Tel. #: Same

Transported to: TGH   Transport Priority: 1

Miles from: 1052.2   To: 1058.8

□ No Transport
REASON:

Billing Information (circle):
Medicare (circled) Medicaid BC/BS
(Indust. Acc.) (circled) Self Other

Subscriber: Joe's Express

Policy #:

Physical Exam

Eye Opening: ☒ Spontaneous ☐ To Pain ☐ To Voice ☐ None

Verbal Response: ☒ Oriented ☐ Confused ☐ Inappropriate ☐ Incomprehensible ☐ None

Motor Response: ☒ Obedience ☐ Purposeful ☐ Withdrawal ☐ Flexion ☐ Extension ☐ None

Skin Condition: ☒ Normal ☐ Cool ☐ Hot ☐ Pale ☐ Flushed ☐ Cyanotic ☐ Diaphoretic

Vital Signs

☐ Unable to Obtain   ☐ Not attempted
REASON:

Time	BP	Pulse	Resp. Rate/Effort
805	132/84	76 Reg.	20 Reg Normal
819	120/90	72	20 Reg Normal
827	90/80	40	24 Reg Normal
831	138/84	60	20 Reg Normal

Allergies: NKA

Current Medications: Diurpress

☒ None ☐ Unknown (Allergies)
☐ None ☐ Unknown (Medications)

Brought with Pt.? ☐ Yes ☒ No

Suspected Diagnosis: ☐ Chronic ☒ Acute
☐ Major Trauma ☐ Acute Medical ☐ Cardiac Arrest ☐ Shock
☐ Minor Trauma ☐ Minor Medical ☒ Cardiac Disorder ☐ ETOH
☐ Soft Tissue Injury ☐ Burns ☐ Ortho ☐ OD/Poison
☐ Neuro ☐ Seizure ☐ Psych ☐ OB/GYN ☐ Neonate

Chief Complaint/History/Changes in Patient Status

49 yo ♂ chest pain
(HPI) while @work unloading a truck experienced ① chest pressure, unable to "catch Breath" and diaphoretic. Presents in No acute Distress, seated on back of Truck. (PMH) HTN (Meds) diurpress NKA (PE) alert/oriented non-diaphoretic BS =/clear. No JVD, ABD soft/non-Tender. Moves all extremities spontaneously. Pain in chest s ↑↓ on Deep Inspire or Palpation. VS - BP 132/84 HR72 NSR secd RR20 Regular/normal (Rx) IV NS, O₂ draw bloods, admin. NitroSpray Pt. states pain @ TNG 3/10, ⓟ TNG 1/10 then 9/10 Note 5 minutes ⓟ Nitro - Pt. c/o Nausea dizziness, becomes pale, Sinus Brady @4/min ③ ectopy BP 90/80. Place Pt-supine ↑NS To wide open, admin. atropine 0.5mg. Rate ↑ To 60/min. Nausea + dizziness dissipate remains ectopy-free. States he "feels better"

Advanced Life Support

Time	/	Medication	/	Rate/Dose	/	Route
0818	/	NS	/	KVO		ⓛ AC/16g 2"
0820	/	TNG	/	0.4mg	/	SL
0827	/	NS	/	Wide	/	IV Infusion
0828	/	Atropine	/	0.5mg	/	IVP
	/		/		/	
	/		/		/	
	/		/		/	

Total Fluid Infused: 500mls

DEFIB: Time:	Time:	Time:	Time:
Joules:	Joules:	Joules:	Joules:

Emergency Care:
☐ CPR ☐ Extricate ☐ Back/Neck Immobilize
☐ Bleed Control ☐ Bandage ☐ Splint ☐ Heat/Cold Applied
☒ O₂ Administration: 4 liters/minute via Nasal
Airway: ☐ Cleared ☐ Oral ☐ Nasal Size: _____ ☐ Suction
Intubate: ☐ Endotracheal ☐ Nasotracheal Size: _____
Assist Ventilation: Rate: _____ Method: _____
☒ ECG Monitor ☒ Rhythm Strip Attached
Transport Position: Semi-fowler To supine

Medical Control: ☐ Direct ☐ C-MED Channel _____
MD# 54   Hospital _____
Hospital Notified Enroute: ☒ Yes ☐ No
☒ C-MED ☐ Dispatcher

Other Response Units/Agencies:

Unit #: P6
EMT/Paramedic Signatures: Paula Karman # 197   John Martix # 188 _____ # _____

Trip#033   page 1 of 2

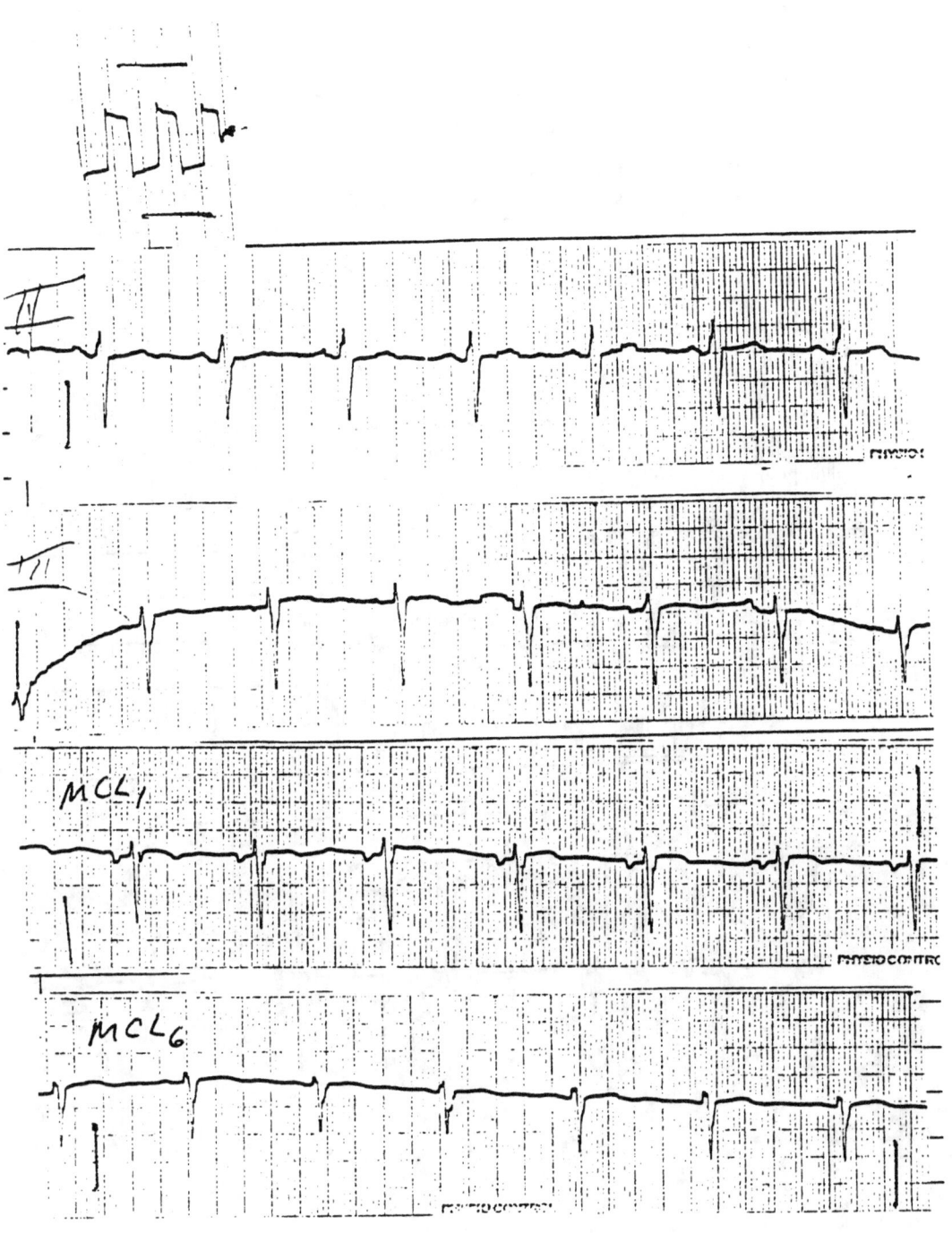

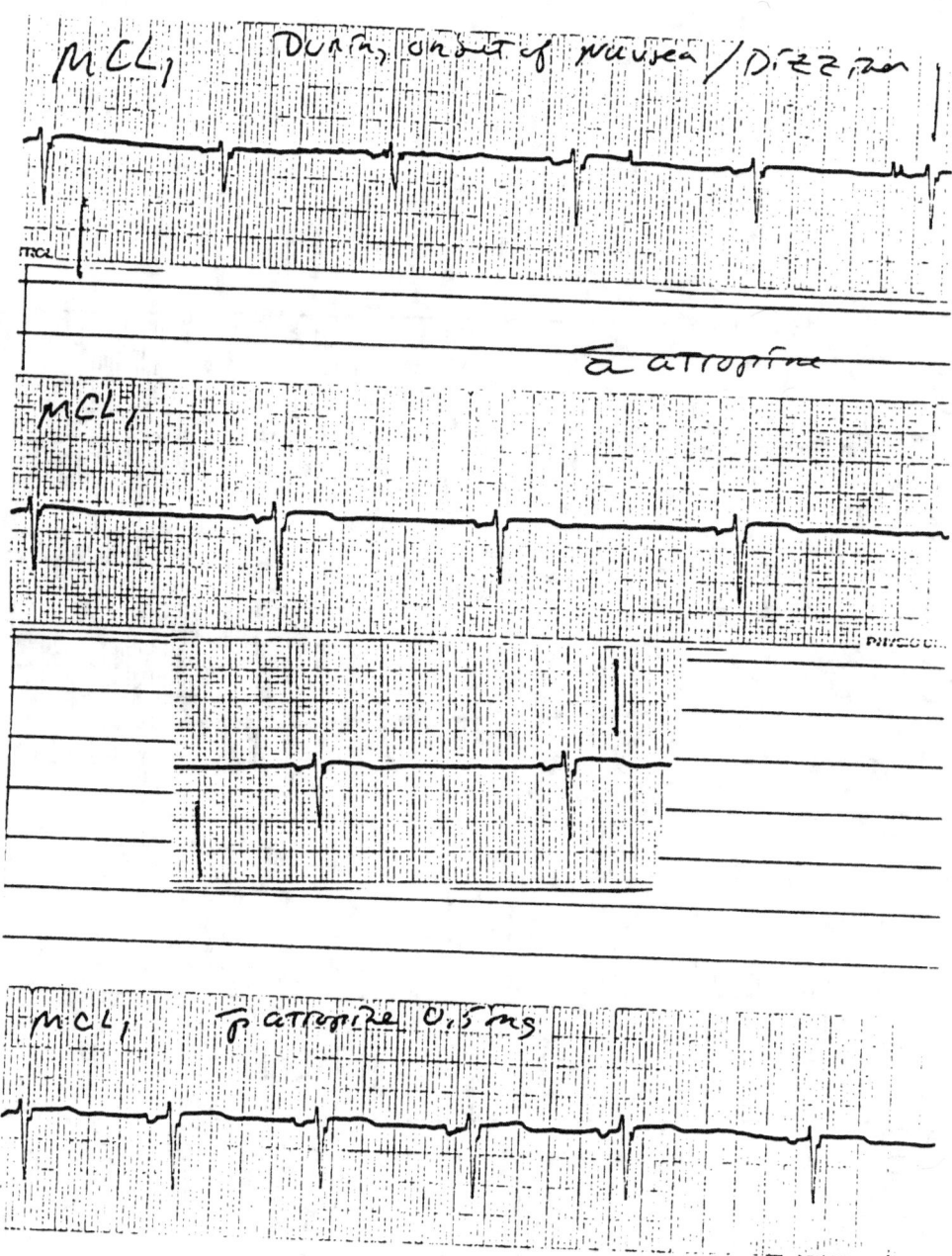

Notes

E.M.S. TRAINING PROGRAM
PATIENT CARE REPORT FORM

© 1992 Kennedy Associates

Patient Name: James Ford	Trip #: 034 Date: 09•30•92
Address: 100 Walker Road	M.R.#: Day: W
Boston MA	Dispatch To: For: Cardiac
DOB: 07-•07-27 Tel. #: 555- 8609	APT 618 on 6th floor
Next of Kin: Richard Ford	Dispatch Time: 716 Arrival Time: 724
Address: 63 Pearce Place	To Hospital: 756 At Hospital: 759
Boston MA	Location at Dispatch:
Relationship: Brother Tel. #: 555-3160	Billing Information (circle):
Transported to: CH Transport Priority:	(Medicare) Medicaid BC/BS
Miles from: To:	Indust. Acc. Self Other
❏ No Transport	Subscriber:
REASON:	
	Policy #:

Physical Exam

Eye Opening (2) ☒ Spontaneous (1) ☒ To Pain   ❏ To Voice   ❏ None

Verbal Response (2) ☒ Oriented (1) ☒ Confused   ❏ Inappropriate   ❏ Incomprehensible   ❏ None

Motor Response (2) ☒ Obedience   ❏ Purposeful (1) ☒ Withdrawal   ❏ Flexion   ❏ Extension   ❏ None

Skin Condition: ❏ Normal   ☒ Cool   ❏ Hot   ☒ Pale   ❏ Flushed   ❏ Cyanotic   ❏ Diaphoretic

Vital Signs

❏ Unable to Obtain   ❏ Not attempted
REASON:

Time	BP	Pulse	Resp. Rate/Effort
7	0	10-20	12
734	0	40-50	12
740	126/74	100	12
752/756	90/60 104/60	100/102	16

Allergies: ❏ None ☒ Unknown

Current Medications: Insulin Dig Ecotrin   ❏ None   ❏ Unknown

Brought with Pt.? ❏ Yes   ❏ No

Suspected Diagnosis: ❏ Chronic ☒ Acute
❏ Major Trauma ❏ Acute Medical ❏ Cardiac Arrest ❏ Shock
❏ Minor Trauma ❏ Minor Medical ☒ Cardiac Disorder ❏ ETOH
❏ Soft Tissue Injury ❏ Burns ❏ Ortho ❏ OD/Poison
❏ Neuro ❏ Seizure ❏ Psych ❏ OB/GYN ❏ Neonate

Emergency Care: ❏ CPR ❏ Extricate ❏ Back/Neck Immobilize
❏ Bleed Control ❏ Bandage ❏ Splint ❏ Heat/Cold Applied
☒ O₂ Administration: 15 liters/minute via NRM
Airway: ❏ Cleared ❏ Oral ❏ Nasal Size: _____ ❏ Suction
Intubate: ❏ Endotracheal ❏ Nasotracheal Size: _____
Assist Ventilation: Rate: _____ Method: _____
☒ ECG Monitor ☒ Rhythm Strip Attached
Transport Position: Trendelenberg

Unit #: P11
EMT/Paramedic Signatures: James Mewl # 165

Chief Complaint/History/Changes in Patient Status

HPI: 65 y/o w ♂ found supine on floor @ home. family member states PMH CABG x4 1 month ago. Diabetic → he experienced an episode of Diarrhea accompanied by Gen weakness @ about 4am → went back to bed → he got up @ 7am → she heard him fell → ? Syncopal episode → found him on floor, hard to arouse → called amb PT Denied SOB, chest pain

PMH CABGx4 1mo. ago. Diabetic Insulin dependent meds Insulin Dig Ecotrin
PE: unresponsive ♂ responding to PNful stimuli ē moans, skin pale cool Dry ECG CHB @ 10-20 ē no peripheral pulses unable to obtain BP B/s clear/= Bilaterally ē no acute distress ⊕ JVD → Idioventricular rate ↑40-50 which is irregular → administered 0.5mg Atropine → NSRE 100 ē 1° Block ē BP 126/74 → PT extricated to vehicle → semi fowlr position in elevator @ which BP 90/60 HR100 → Placed Trendelenberg BP 104/60 HR100 ↑↑ ms ↑ ēBP/HR CA+Ox3

Advanced Life Support

Time	Medication	Rate/Dose	Route
736	NS	500 cc Bolus 16g 1½"	Ⓛ AC
738	LR	wide 700 cc 16g 1½"	Ⓛ AC
740	Atropine	0.5 mg	IVP
757	NS	500 cc Bolus	IV
	/	/	
	/	/	
	/	/	

Total Fluid Infused: 1700 mls

DEFIB: Time: Time: Time: Time:
Joules: Joules: Joules: Joules:

Medical Control: ❏ Direct ❏ C-MED Channel _____
MD# _____   Hospital _____
Hospital Notified Enroute: ☒ Yes ❏ No
☒ C-MED ❏ Dispatcher

Other Response Units/Agencies:

Trip#034 page 1 of 3

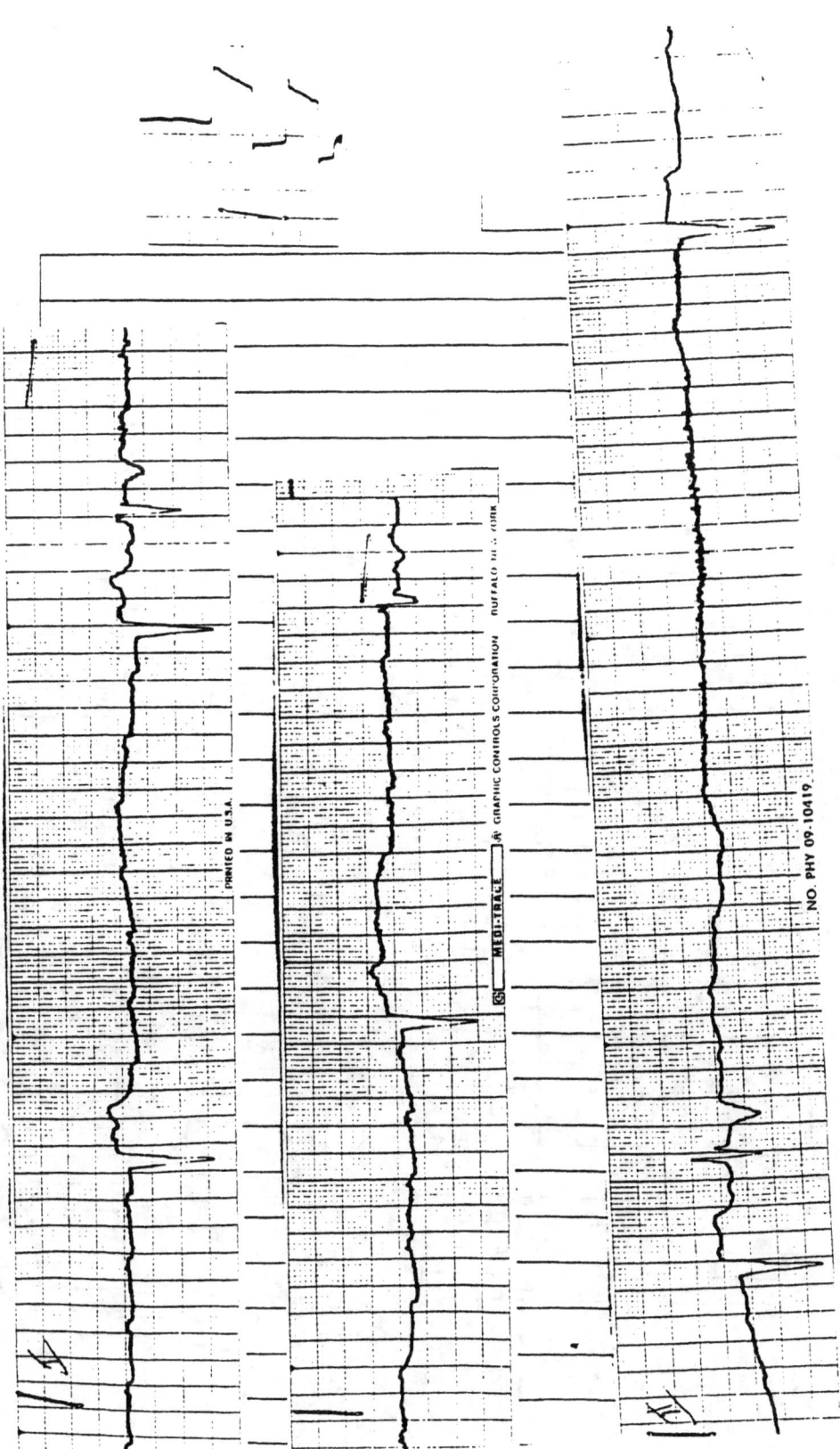

Trip #034 page 2 of 3

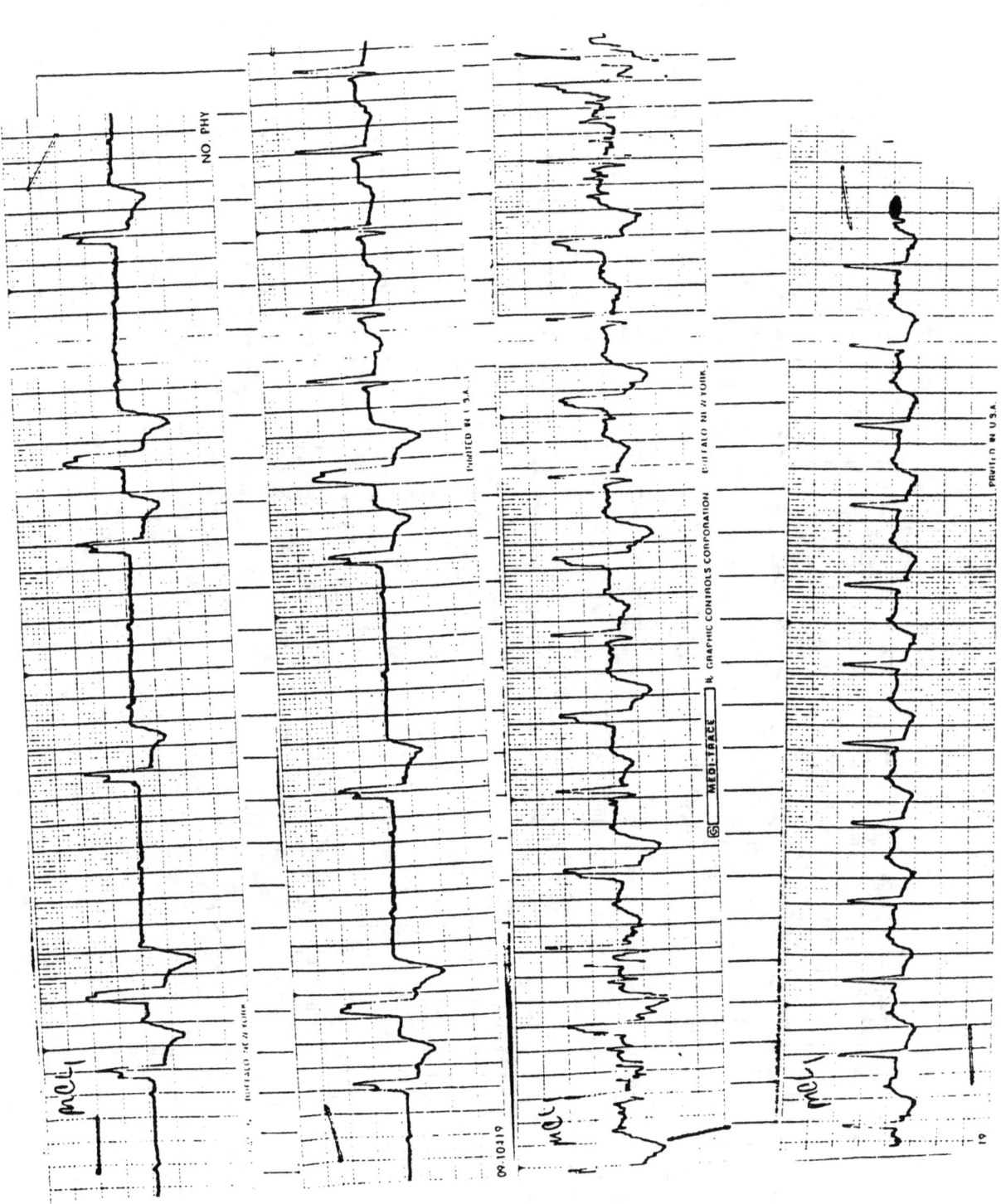

Trip # 034 page 3 of 3

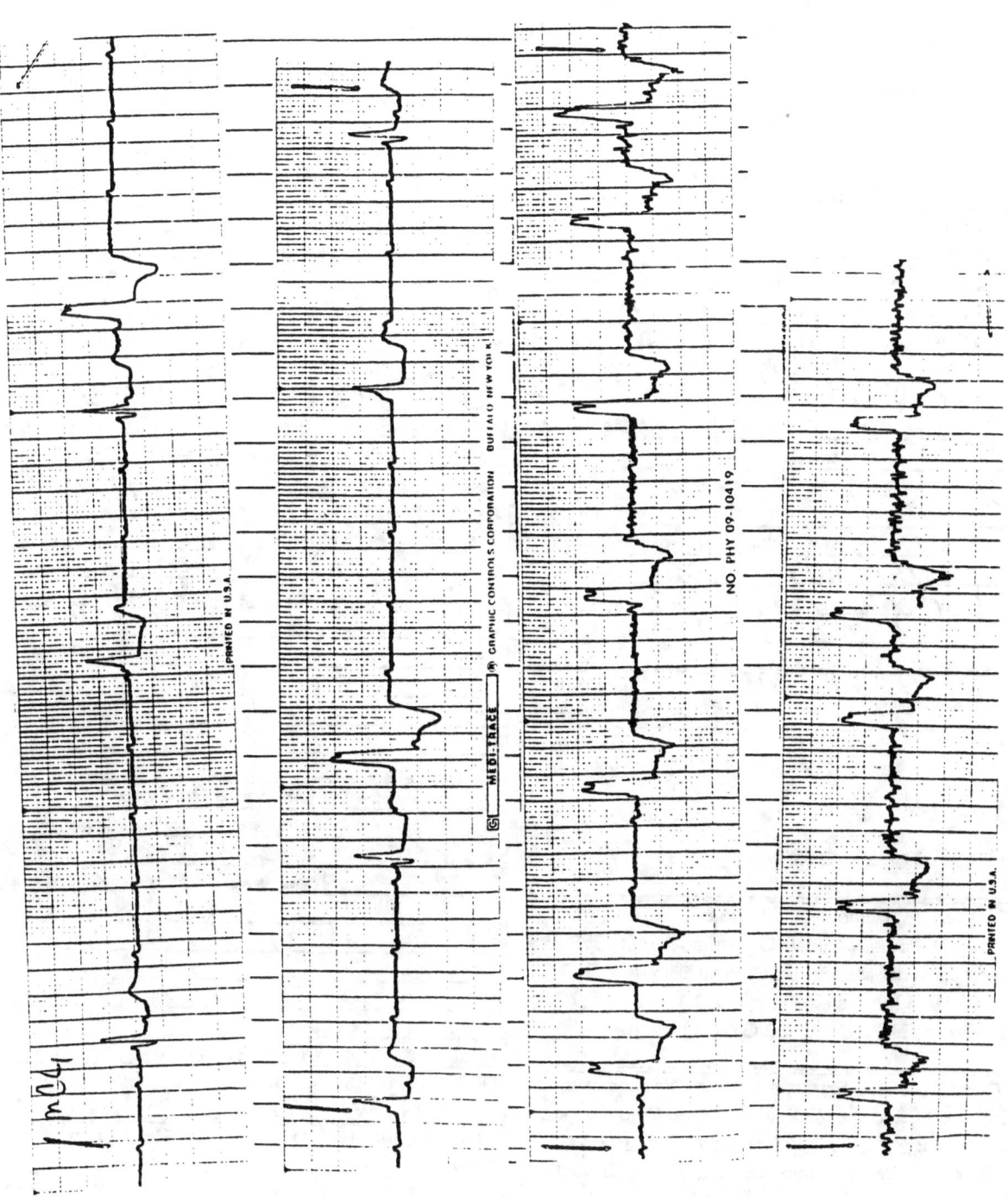

E.M.S. TRAINING PROGRAM
PATIENT CARE REPORT FORM

© 1992 Kennedy Associates

Patient Name: Robert Greene	Trip #: 035 Date: Sept. 30, 1992
Address: 68 South Blvd	M.R.#: Day: Wednesday
Boston MA	Dispatch To: Heart For:
DOB: Jan. 16, 1926 Tel. #:	APT. 38 3rd floor
Next of Kin:	Dispatch Time: 1819 Arrival Time: 1826
Address:	To Hospital: 1844 At Hospital: 1852
	Location at Dispatch:
Relationship: Tel. #:	Billing Information (circle):
Transported to: Community Transport Priority:	(Medicare) Medicaid BC/BS
Miles from: To:	Indust. Acc. Self Other
❏ No Transport	Subscriber:
REASON:	
	Policy #: 041 628056A

Physical Exam

Eye Opening	☒ Spontaneous	❏ To Pain
	❏ To Voice	❏ None
Verbal Response	☒ Oriented	❏ Confused
	❏ Inappropriate	❏ Incomprehensible ❏ None
Motor Response	☒ Obedience	❏ Purposeful ❏ Withdrawal
	❏ Flexion	❏ Extension ❏ None
Skin Condition	❏ Normal ❏ Cool ❏ Hot ❏ Pale slight	
	❏ Flushed ❏ Cyanotic ☒ Diaphoretic	

Vital Signs

❏ Unable to Obtain   ❏ Not attempted
REASON:

Time	BP	Pulse	Resp. Rate/Effort
1830	138/66	140	24
1852	118/60	140	28

Allergies: ❏ None
                          ❏ Unknown

Current Medications: ❏ None
                          ❏ Unknown

Brought with Pt.?   ❏ Yes   ❏ No

Suspected Diagnosis: ☒ Chronic ☒ Acute
❏ Major Trauma ☒ Acute Medical ❏ Cardiac Arrest ❏ Shock
❏ Minor Trauma ❏ Minor Medical ❏ Cardiac Disorder ❏ ETOH
❏ Soft Tissue Injury ❏ Burns ❏ Ortho ❏ OD/Poison
❏ Neuro ❏ Seizure ❏ Psych ❏ OB/GYN ❏ Neonate

Emergency Care: ❏ CPR ❏ Extricate ❏ Back/Neck Immobilize
❏ Bleed Control ❏ Bandage ❏ Splint ❏ Heat/Cold Applied
☒ O₂ Administration: __6__ liters/minute via **Nebulizer**
Airway: ❏ Cleared ❏ Oral ❏ Nasal Size: _____ ❏ Suction
Intubate: ❏ Endotracheal ❏ Nasotracheal Size: _____
Assist Ventilation: Rate: _____ Method: _____
☒ ECG Monitor ☒ Rhythm Strip Attached
Transport Position: Fowlers

Unit #: P5   EMT/Paramedic Signatures:
E. Carlson   #

Chief Complaint/History/Changes in Patient Status

72 y o m complains of 1 Hour of S.O.B with coughing. He is in mild to moderate distress consc alert or x3 skin warm moist No JVD chest BS= fine rales all over (L) and scattered wheezing over (R) PT has trace of pedal edema.
ECG - A-flutter with 2:1 conduction PMH COPD seen all day today at Hosp and released. He had a few hours of relief before symptoms Reoccurred. meds digoxin, Halcion, Bactrim, atrovent, ventolin
treatment O₂, Albuterol + IV D5W at TKO with some relief

Advanced Life Support

Time	/	Medication	/	Rate/Dose	/	Route
1835	/	D5W		TKO (500ml)	18 (g)	hand
1838	/	Albuterol		1.5mls / 2.5saline		mask
	/		/		/	
	/		/		/	
	/		/		/	
	/		/		/	
	/		/		/	

Total Fluid Infused: @ 10 mls

DEFIB: Time:	Time:	Time:	Time:
Joules:	Joules:	Joules:	Joules:

Medical Control: ❏ Direct ❏ C-MED Channel _____
MD# _____   Hospital _____
Hospital Notified Enroute: ❏ Yes   ❏ No
                               ❏ C-MED ❏ Dispatcher

Other Response Units/Agencies:

Trip # 035

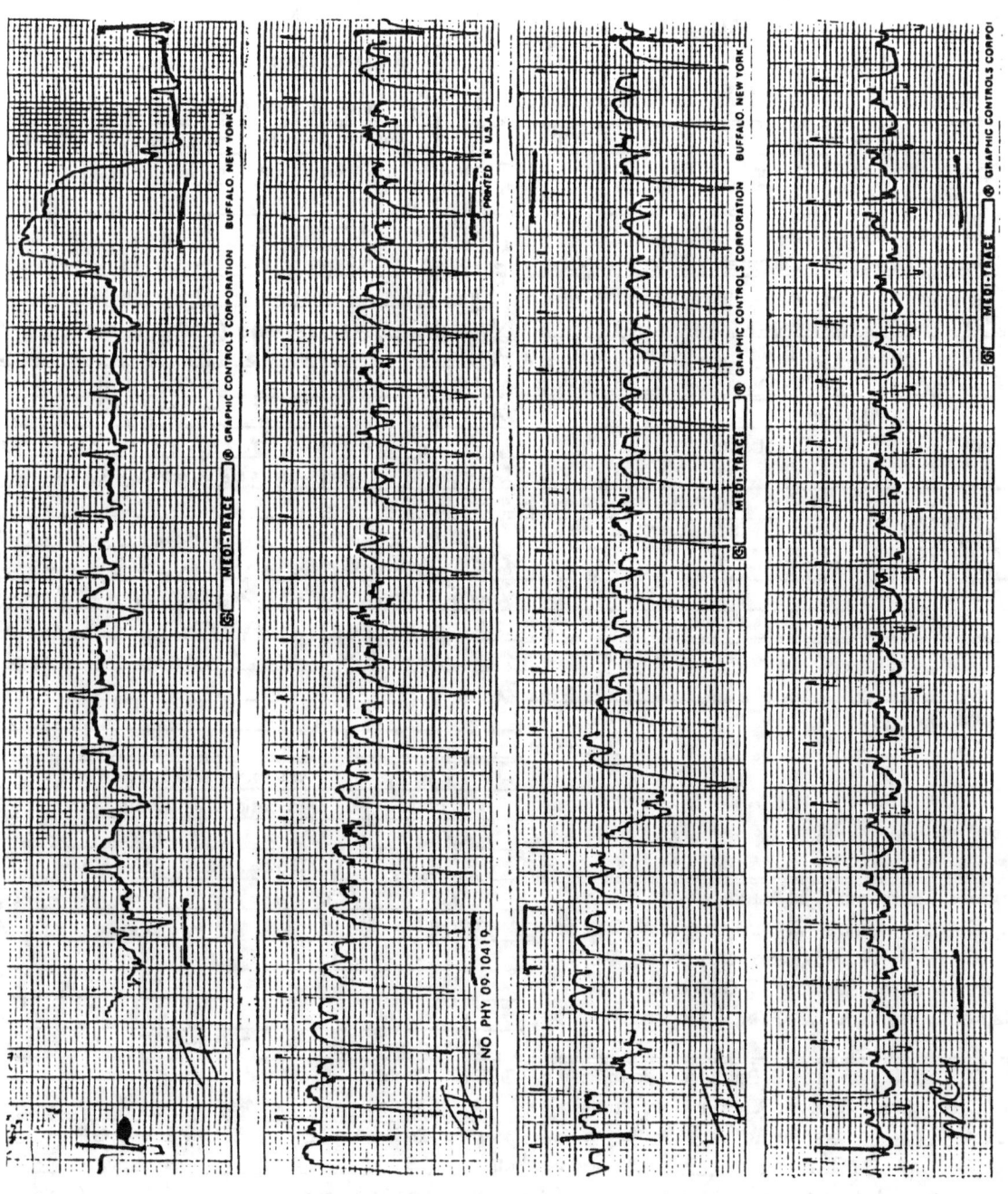

E.M.S. TRAINING PROGRAM
PATIENT CARE REPORT FORM

© 1992 Kennedy Associat

Patient Name: Paul Hendy	Trip #: 036	Date: 9/30/92
Address: 1058 W 4th Ave	M.R.#:	Day: Wed.
Washington DC	Dispatch To: airport	For: cardiac
DOB: 10/28/13 Tel. #: 555-7139		
Next of Kin: Joan	Dispatch Time: 1312	Arrival Time: 1324
Address: S/A	To Hospital: 1335	At Hospital: 1346

Location at Dispatch:

Relationship: Wife   Tel. #:

Transported to: Trauma Center.   Transport Priority: 1
Miles from: 12564   To: 12580

❏ No Transport
REASON:

Billing Information (circle): **(Medicare)** Medicaid BC/BS
Indust. Acc. Self Other

Subscriber: Patient

Policy #: Not Available

Physical Exam

Eye Opening	☒ Spontaneous ❏ To Pain	
	❏ To Voice ❏ None	
Verbal Response	☒ Oriented ❏ Confused	
	❏ Inappropriate ❏ Incomprehensible ❏ None	
Motor Response	☒ Obedience ❏ Purposeful ❏ Withdrawal	
	❏ Flexion ❏ Extension ❏ None	
Skin Condition	❏ Normal ❏ Cool ❏ Hot ❏ Pale	
	❏ Flushed ❏ Cyanotic ☒ Diaphoretic	

Vital Signs

❏ Unable to Obtain   ❏ Not attempted
REASON:

Time	BP	Pulse	Resp. Rate/Effort
BLS @ 1320	102/P	—	20 Reg
1340	110/P	240	20 Reg/full

Allergies: N KA   ☒ None ❏ Unknown

Current Medications: denies   ☒ None ❏ Unknown

Brought with Pt.? ❏ Yes ❏ No

Suspected Diagnosis: ❏ Chronic ☒ Acute
❏ Major Trauma ❏ Acute Medical ❏ Cardiac Arrest ❏ Shock
❏ Minor Trauma ❏ Minor Medical ☒ Cardiac Disorder ❏ ETOH
❏ Soft Tissue Injury ❏ Burns ❏ Ortho ❏ OD/Poison
❏ Neuro ❏ Seizure ❏ Psych ❏ OB/GYN ❏ Neonate

Emergency Care: ❏ CPR ❏ Extricate ❏ Back/Neck Immobilize
❏ Bleed Control ❏ Bandage ❏ Splint ❏ Heat/Cold Applied
☒ O₂ Administration: 15 liters/minute via Non-Rebreath.
Airway: ❏ Cleared ❏ Oral ❏ Nasal Size: _____ ❏ Suction
Intubate: ❏ Endotracheal ❏ Nasotracheal Size: _____
Assist Ventilation: Rate: _____ Method: _____
☒ ECG Monitor ☒ Rhythm Strip Attached
Transport Position: Semi-fowler

Unit # 78

Chief Complaint/History/Changes in Patient Status

78 y/o ♂ (CC) chest pain episode c̄ irregular heartbeat
(HPI) on airplane - 2 periods of chest pain during flight. Currently pain-free. Presents in rear of BLS Ambulance.
(PMH) M.I. x 20 yrs ago (meds) none (NKA)
(PE) alert/oriented 2+ diaphoretic
No JVD BS =/clear ABD soft non-tender
Weighs aprox 70 kg ECG Runs of V-T lasting aprox 6 seconds each c̄ Sinus Beats (2) interposed between runs of V.T. Is pain-free.
(Rx) IV NS KVO, Draw Bloods, maintaining ??
↑ Flow Non-Rebreather begun by EMT's.
begin Transport. Administer Lidocaine 70?
Slows duration of V-T. Begin Lidocaine Infusion 2mg/min. Repeat Lidocaine 70 mg
Bolus - Abolish V-T as arriving at Hospital

Advanced Life Support

Time	Medication	Rate/Dose	Route
1332	NS	KVO	@ Ac 18, 16
1336	Lidocaine	70 mg	IVP
1338	Lidocaine	2mg/min	IV Infusion
1342	Lidocaine	70 mg	IVP

Total Fluid Infused: < 50 mls

DEFIB: Time:	Time:	Time:	Time:
Joules:	Joules:	Joules:	Joules:

Medical Control: ❏ Direct ❏ C-MED Channel _____
MD# _____   Hospital _____
Hospital Notified Enroute: ❏ Yes ❏ No
❏ C-MED ❏ Dispatcher

Other Response Units/Agencies:

EMT/Paramedic Signatures:
M.Kelly # 170   P. Harbor # 172   # _____

Trip #036   page 1 of 5

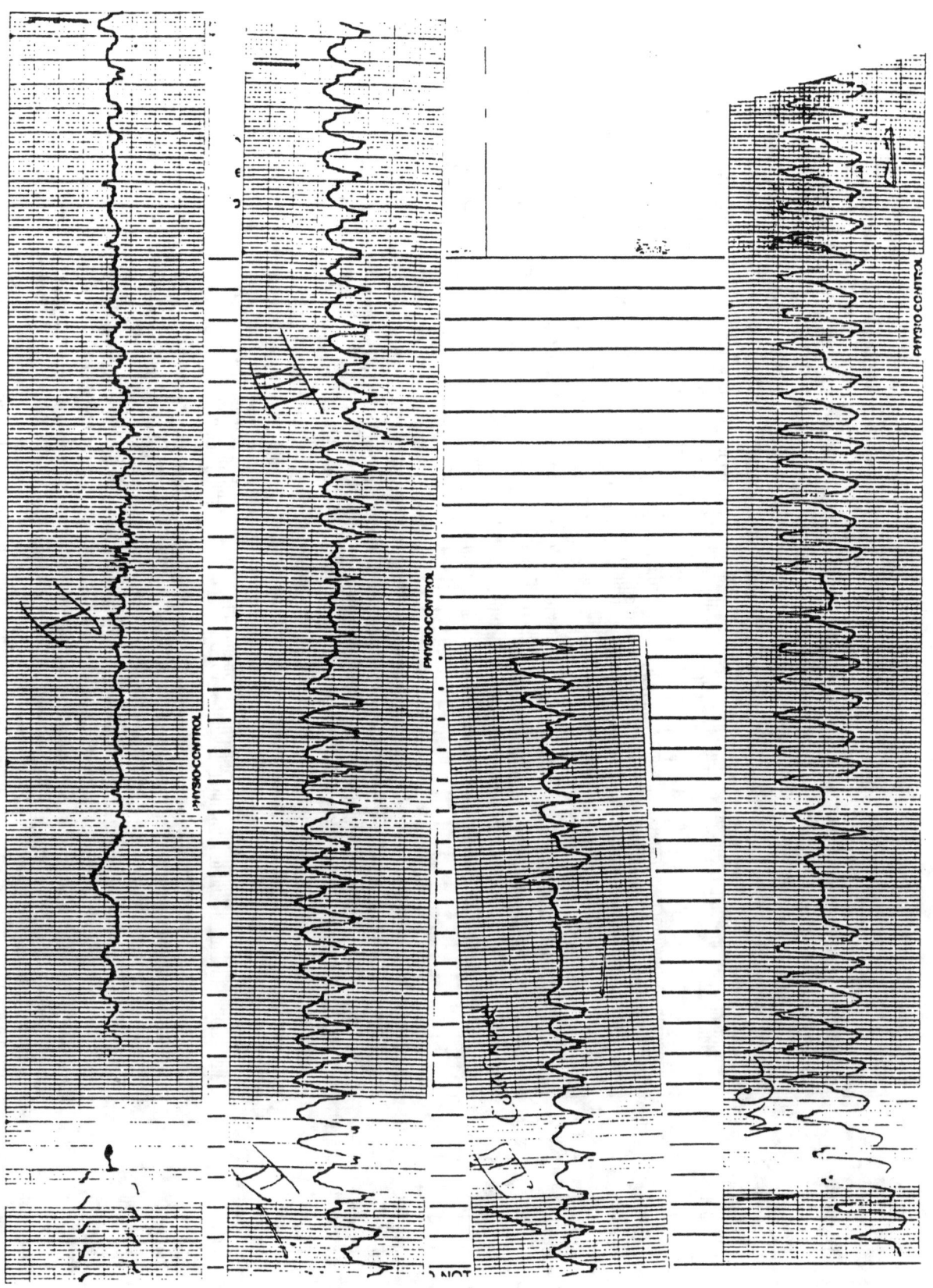

Trip #036   page 2 of 5

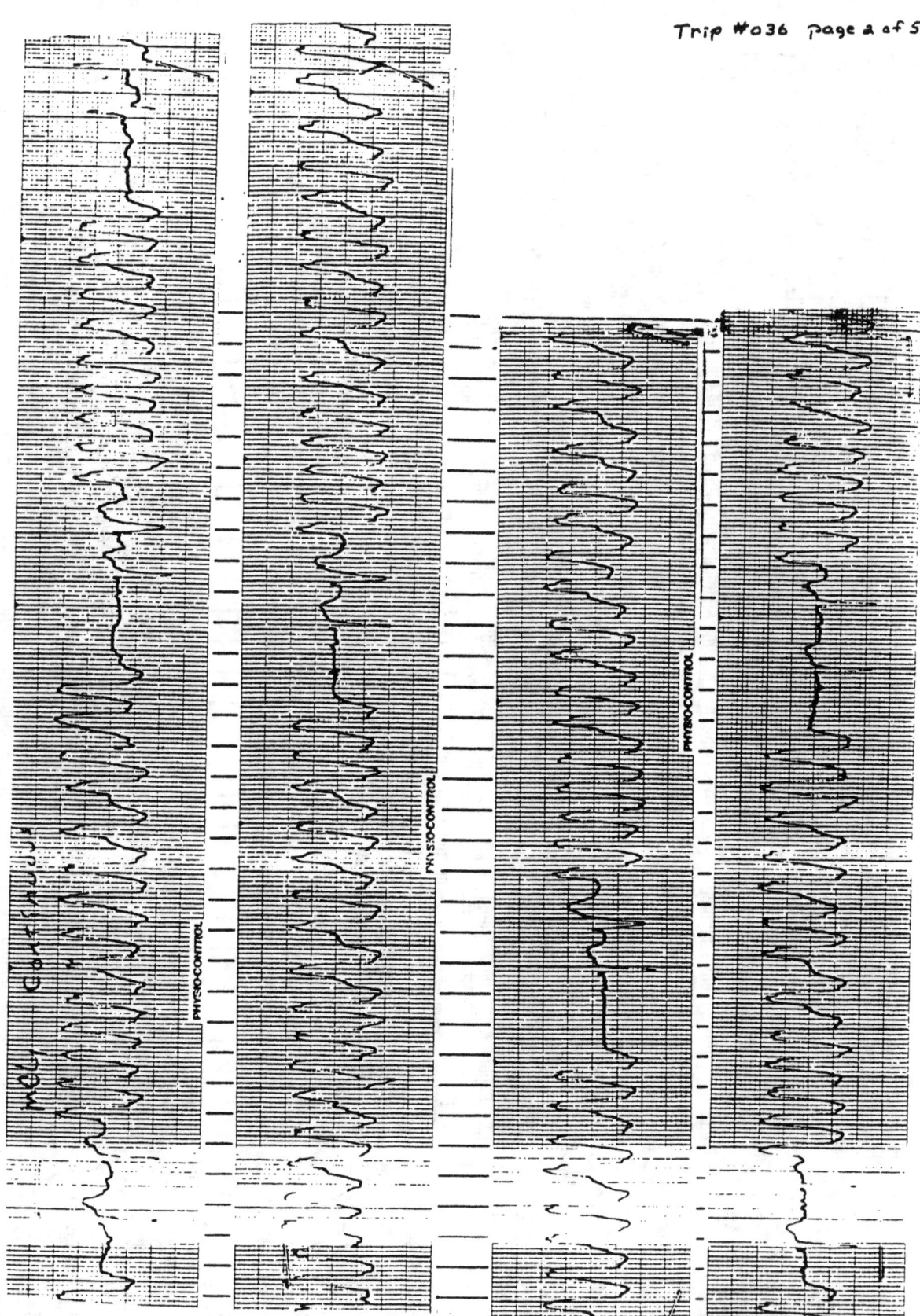

Trip #036 page 3 of 5

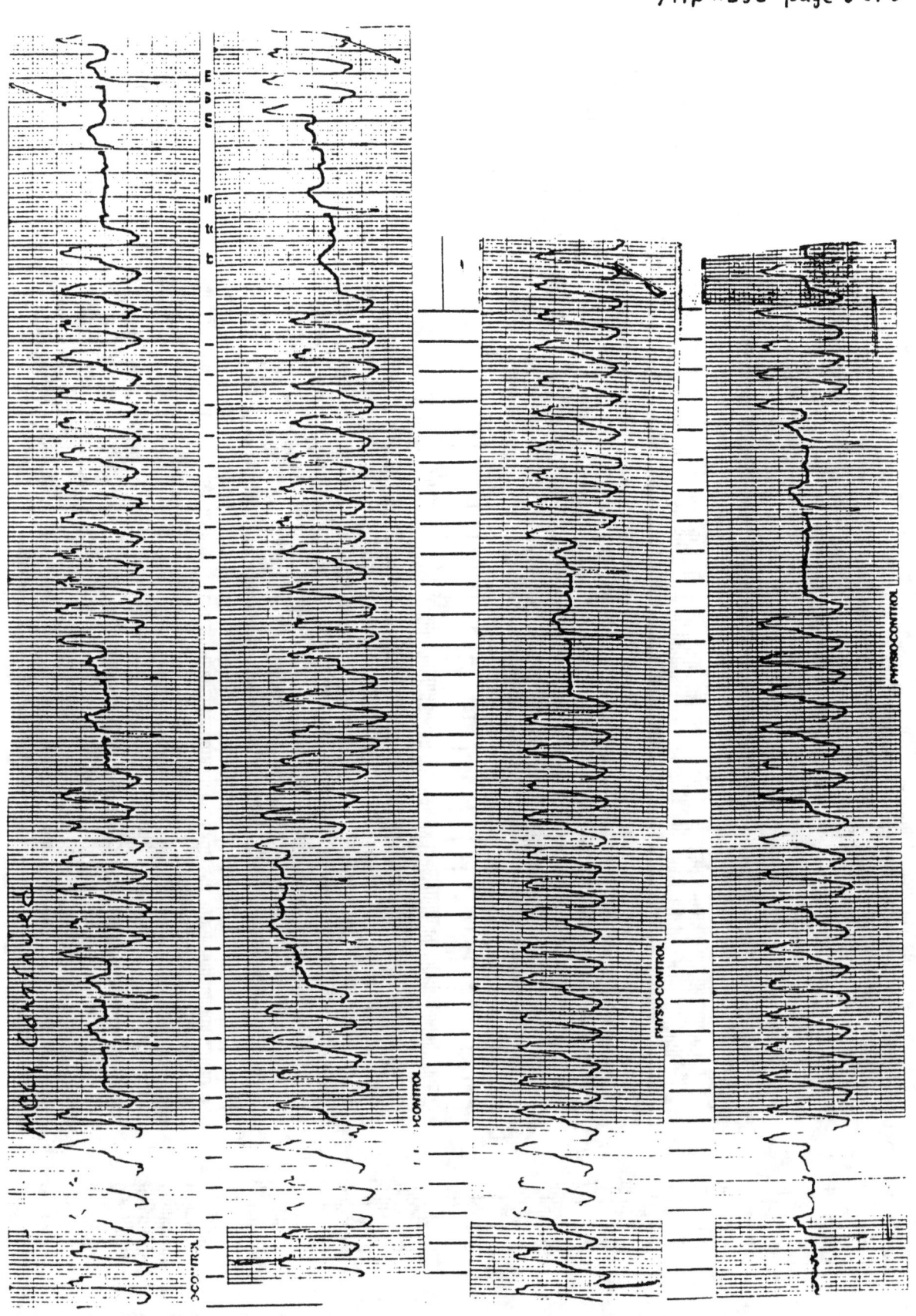

Trip #036 page 4 of 5

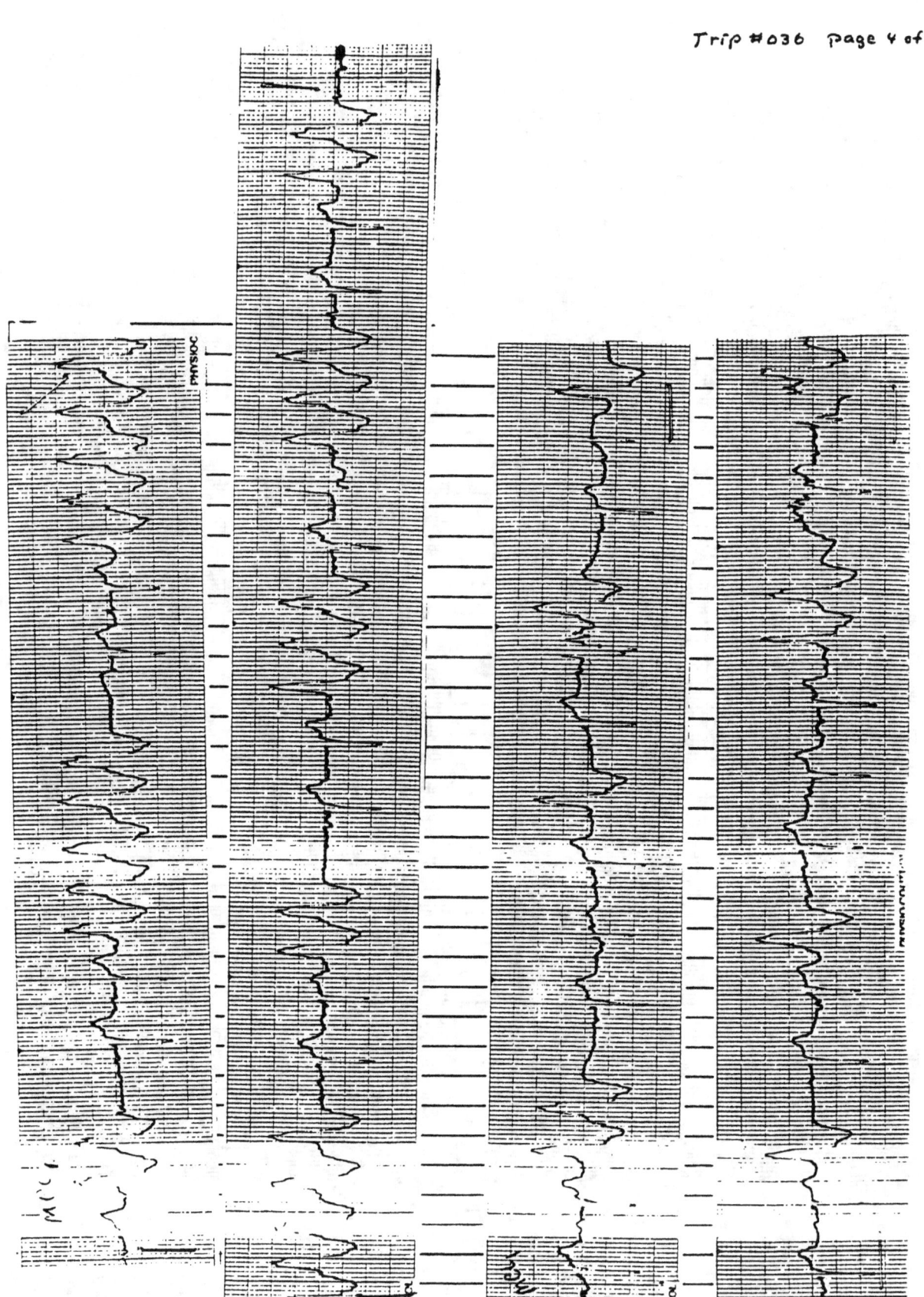

Trip #036 page 5 of 5

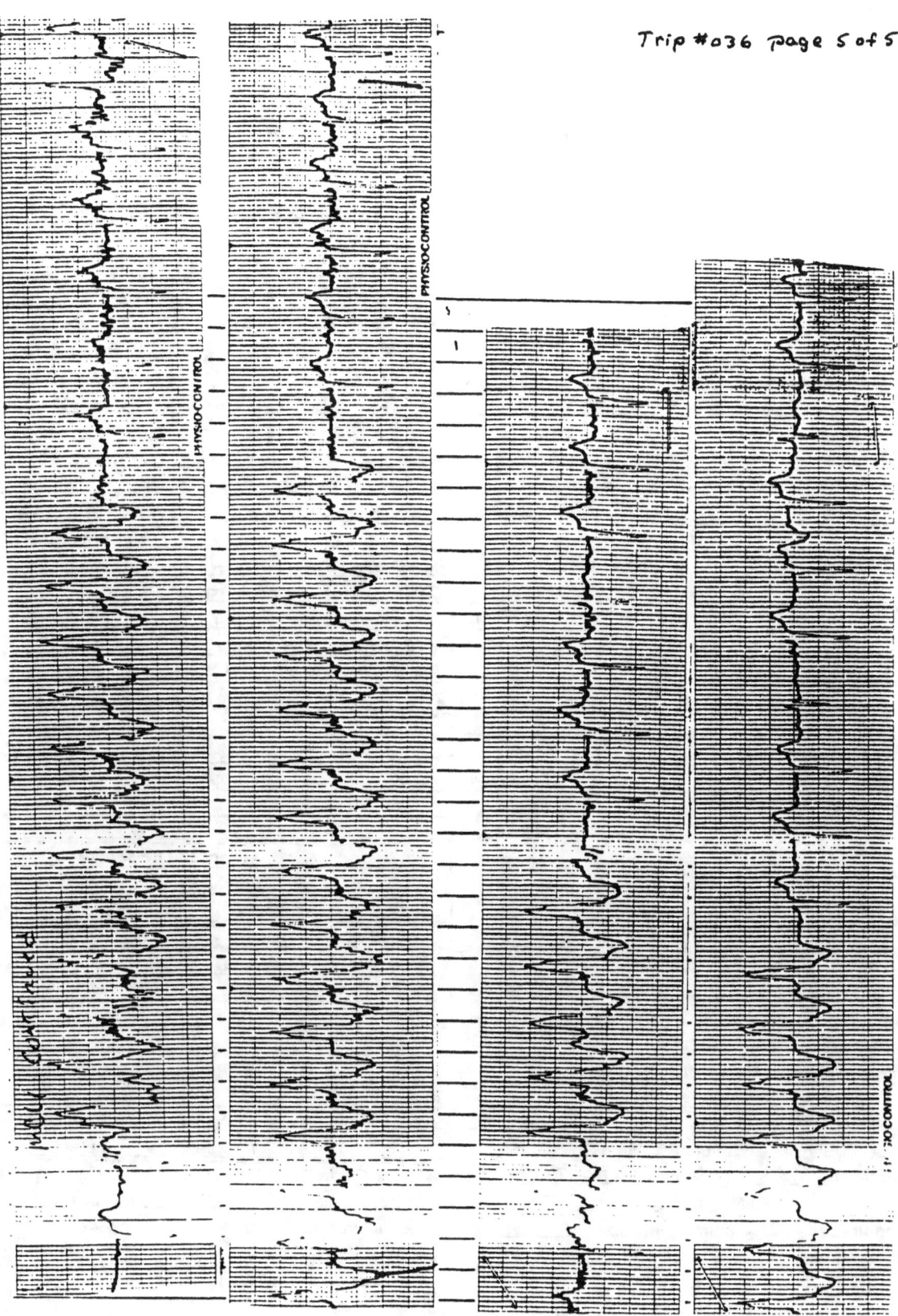

E.M.S. TRAINING PROGRAM
PATIENT CARE REPORT FORM

© 1992 Kennedy Associates

Patient Name: David Jackson	Trip #: 037 — Date: 9/30/92
Address: 149 Regency Blvd, Boston MA	M.R.#: — Day: WED.
DOB: 11-02-07 — Tel. #: 555-4237	Dispatch To: — For:
Next of Kin: David Jackson Sr	Dispatch Time: 1100 — Arrival Time: 1105
Address: 45 Walnut Way, Boston MA	To Hospital: 1122 — At Hospital: 1128
Relationship: Son — Tel. #: 555-2725	Location at Dispatch:
Transported to: Trauma Gen. Hosp — Transport Priority:	Billing Information (circle):
Miles from: 16450 — T66455 — 1	(Medicare) Medicaid BC/BS
❑ No Transport	Indust. Acc. Self Other J medos
REASON:	Subscriber: Patient
	Policy #: 201 60 4096A

Physical Exam

Eye Opening: ☒ Spontaneous ❑ To Pain ❑ To Voice ❑ None

Verbal Response: ☒ Oriented ❑ Confused ❑ Inappropriate ❑ Incomprehensible ❑ None

Motor Response: ☒ Obedience ❑ Purposeful ❑ Withdrawal ❑ Flexion ❑ Extension ❑ None

Skin Condition: ❑ Normal ❑ Cool ❑ Hot ☒ Pale ❑ Flushed ❑ Cyanotic ☒ Diaphoretic

Vital Signs

❑ Unable to Obtain   ❑ Not attempted
REASON:

Time	BP	Pulse	Resp. Rate/Effort
1105	150/90	150	36 labored

Allergies: NKA   ☒ None ❑ Unknown

Current Medications: See Note →   ❑ None ❑ Unknown

Brought with Pt.? ❑ Yes ❑ No

Suspected Diagnosis: ❑ Chronic ☒ Acute
❑ Major Trauma ☒ Acute Medical ❑ Cardiac Arrest ❑ Shock
❑ Minor Trauma ❑ Minor Medical ☒ Cardiac Disorder ❑ ETOH
❑ Soft Tissue Injury ❑ Burns ❑ Ortho ❑ OD/Poison
❑ Neuro ❑ Seizure ❑ Psych ❑ OB/GYN ❑ Neonate

Emergency Care: ❑ CPR ☒ Extricate ❑ Back/Neck Immobilize
❑ Bleed Control ❑ Bandage ❑ Splint ❑ Heat/Cold Applied
☒ O₂ Administration: 15 liters/minute via Non-Rebreather
Airway: ❑ Cleared ❑ Oral ❑ Nasal Size: _____ ❑ Suction
Intubate: ❑ Endotracheal ❑ Nasotracheal Size: _____
Assist Ventilation: Rate: _____ Method: _____
❑ ECG Monitor ❑ Rhythm Strip Attached
Transport Position: Upright on Stretcher

Chief Complaint/History/Changes in Patient Status

84yo ♂ Dyspnea c̄ chest Pain
(HPI) apparent ↑ Dyspnea x 8days presents in a health center clinic on BLS Stretcher c̄ IV/ECG. Is non-English speaking (speaks Russ.
(PMH) Hypertension, Diabetes (NKA)
(meds) HCTZ + Diazide, Alupent, Yohimbine, Nizoral, Hydrocortisone, menthol lotion, Erythromycin, Haloprogin, HydraQuinone.
(PE) alert/oriented as determined through interpreter. Pale, diaphoretic, No prominent JVD c̄ Bilateral Rales bases to apices and Bilateral pedal edema. ECG Sinus Tach @ 150/min c̄ frequent PAC's BP 150/90 RR 36 labored ABD appears non-tender.
(Rx) ↑ FiO₂ (non-Rebreather) IV D₅W KVO administer NTG 0.4mg SL + Lasix 40mg IVP all during Transport. arrive @ Hospital at end of Lasix administration.

Advanced Life Support

Time	Medication	Rate/Dose	Route
1123	D₅W	KVO	(L) Thumb 22g
1126	NTG	0.4mg	SL
1127	Lasix	40mg	IVP

Total Fluid Infused: < 50 mls

DEFIB: Time:	Time:	Time:	Time:
Joules:	Joules:	Joules:	Joules:

Medical Control: ❑ Direct ❑ C-MED Channel _____
MD# 40   Hospital _____
Hospital Notified Enroute: ❑ Yes ❑ No ❑ C-MED ❑ Dispatcher

Other Response Units/Agencies:

Unit # P12   EMT/Paramedic Signatures: Mary Dool # 183   Harris # 189   # _____

Trip #037

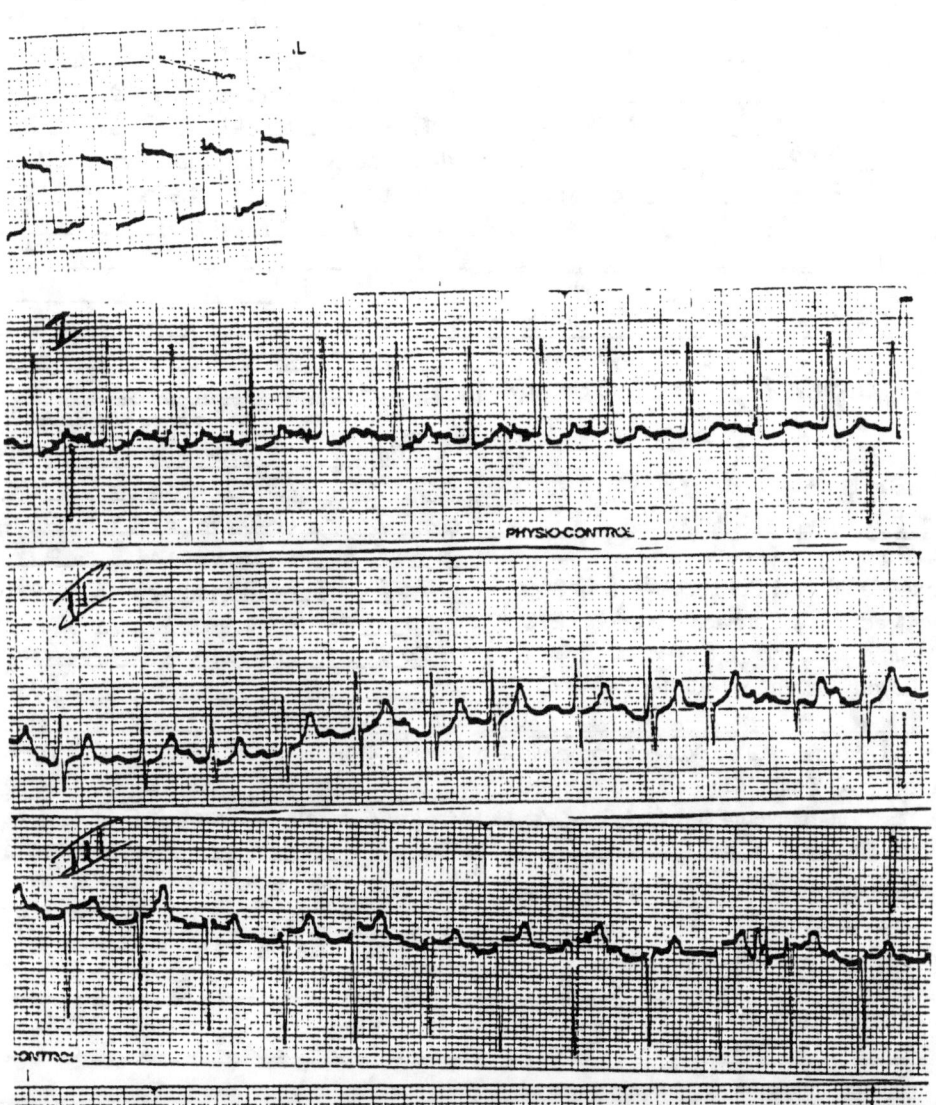

E.M.S. TRAINING PROGRAM
PATIENT CARE REPORT FORM

© 1992 Kennedy Associate

Patient Name: John Joyce	Trip #: 038 Date: Sept. 30, 1992
Address: 580 Independence Ave	M.R.#: Day: Wednesday
Boston MA	Dispatch To: For: O.D.
DOB: May 28, 1925 Tel. #: 555-3871	Apartment #250 - 25th floor
Next of Kin:	Dispatch Time: 0715 Arrival Time: 0724
Address:	To Hospital: 0809 At Hospital: 0813
	Location at Dispatch: Quarters
Relationship: Tel. #:	Billing Information (circle):
Transported to: T G H Transport Priority: 1	Medicare Medicaid BC/BS
Miles from: To:	Indust. Acc. Self Other
☐ No Transport	Subscriber:
REASON:	
	Policy #:

Physical Exam

Eye Opening	☒ Spontaneous	☐ To Pain
	☐ To Voice	☐ None
Verbal Response	☒ Oriented	☐ Confused
	☐ Inappropriate	☐ Incomprehensible ☐ None
Motor Response	☒ Obedience	☐ Purposeful ☐ Withdrawal
	☐ Flexion	☐ Extension ☐ None
Skin Condition	☒ Normal ☐ Cool ☐ Hot ☐ Pale	
	☐ Flushed ☐ Cyanotic ☐ Diaphoretic	

Vital Signs

☐ Unable to Obtain   ☐ Not attempted
REASON:

Time	BP	Pulse	Resp. Rate/Effort
0730	120/80	270	18 Regular/normal
0755	78/P	240	20 Regular/Normal
0810	80/50	220	18 Regular/normal

Allergies: STATES NKDA   ☐ None ☐ Unknown

Current Medications: LISTED IN REPORT ↗   ☐ None ☐ Unknown

Brought with Pt.?   ☐ Yes ☒ No

Suspected Diagnosis: ☐ Chronic   ☒ Acute
☐ Major Trauma ☐ Acute Medical ☐ Cardiac Arrest ☐ Shock
☐ Minor Trauma ☐ Minor Medical ☒ Cardiac Disorder ☐ ETOH
☐ Soft Tissue Injury ☐ Burns ☐ Ortho ☒ OD/Poison
☐ Neuro ☐ Seizure ☐ Psych ☐ OB/GYN ☐ Neonate

Emergency Care: ☐ CPR ☐ Extricate ☐ Back/Neck Immobilize
☐ Bleed Control ☐ Bandage ☐ Splint ☐ Heat/Cold Applied
☒ O₂ Administration: 4 liters/minute via Nasal Cannula
Airway: ☐ Cleared ☐ Oral ☐ Nasal Size: ☐ Suction
Intubate: ☐ Endotracheal ☐ Nasotracheal Size:
Assist Ventilation: Rate: Method:
☒ ECG Monitor ☒ Rhythm Strip Attached
Transport Position: fowler

Unit # P3   EMT/Paramedic Signatures:
176   # 179

Chief Complaint/History/Changes in Patient Status

67 yo↗ who allegedly ingested ~30 (30mg) MS about 1 hour ā arrival of EMS. Found sitti cons & A C/O Back pain only PE: Good color warm & Dry No JVD BP 120/80 P 260 SVT R18 Clear/Equal Bilaterally PMH: COPD Bone & Prostate CA Rx Theodur compazi Oxycodone MS   Pt Given IV D5W initiated Kl Adenocard 6mg Given IV s̄ Δ, Adenocard 12mg Given IV ē Brief To a MAT at 160. 2nd administration of Adenocard 12mg IV AGAin results in Transient Δ TO MAT at 180 then in SVT @ 240. Pt. Given CaCl 500mg slow IV followed by Verapamil 5mg IV ē ECG alternat between on SVT & an MAT vs. A F ē BP 80/ on arrival at Hospital

Advanced Life Support

Time	Medication	Rate/Dose	Route
0740	D5W 500	TKO	⁴/₈ angio ®fo
0742	Adenocard	6 mg	IVP
0748	Adenocard	12 mg	IVP
0755	Adenocard	12 mg	IVP
0800	CaCl	500 mg	Slow IV
0805	Verapamil	5 mg	IV

Total Fluid Infused: TKO < 50 mls

DEFIB: Time:	Time:	Time:	Time:
Joules:	Joules:	Joules:	Joules:

Medical Control: ☐ Direct ☒ C-MED Channel 3
MD# 24   Hospital
Hospital Notified Enroute: ☒ Yes ☐ No
☒ C-MED ☐ Dispatcher

Other Response Units/Agencies:
A4

Trip # 038   page 1 of 3

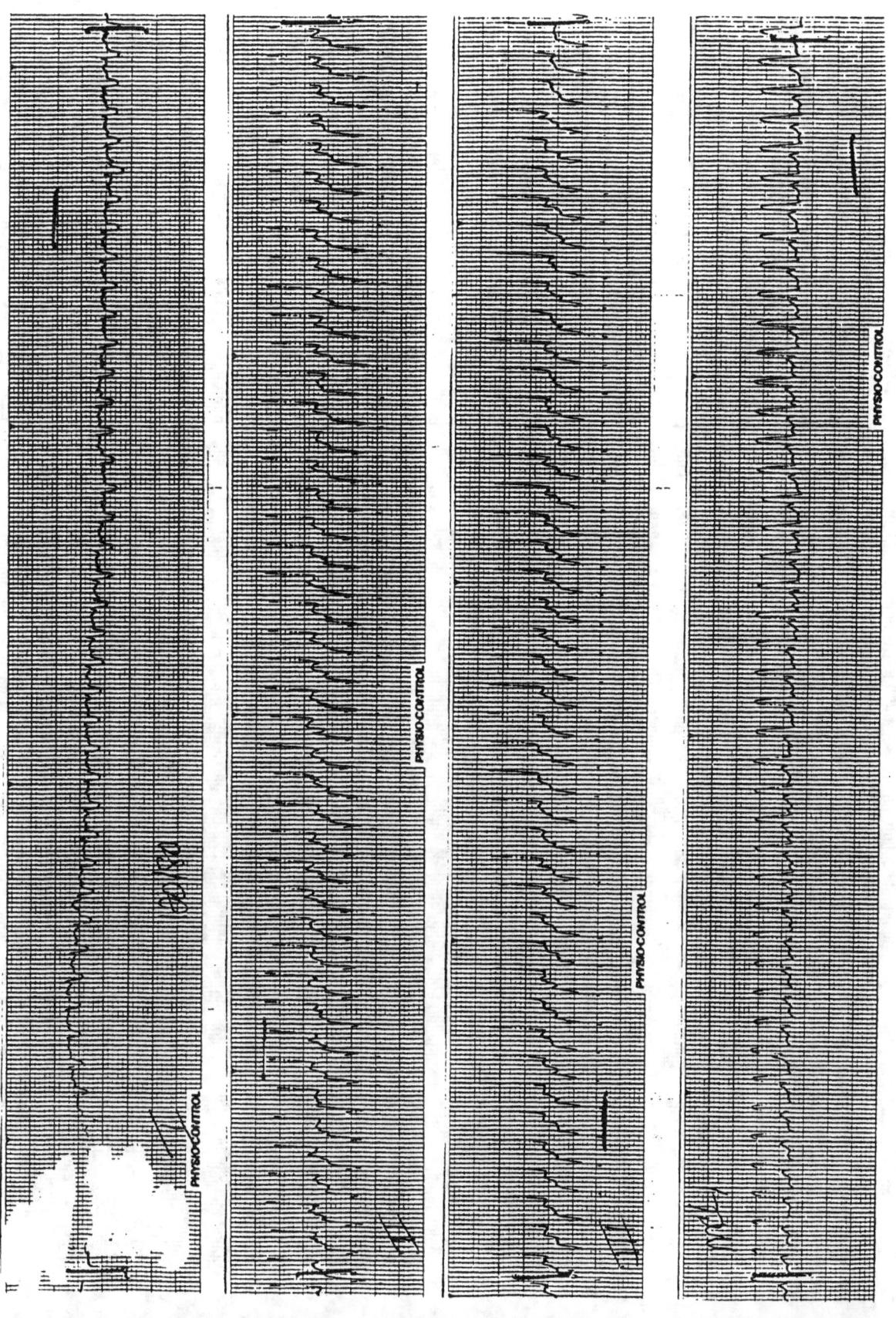

Trip #038 page 2 of 3

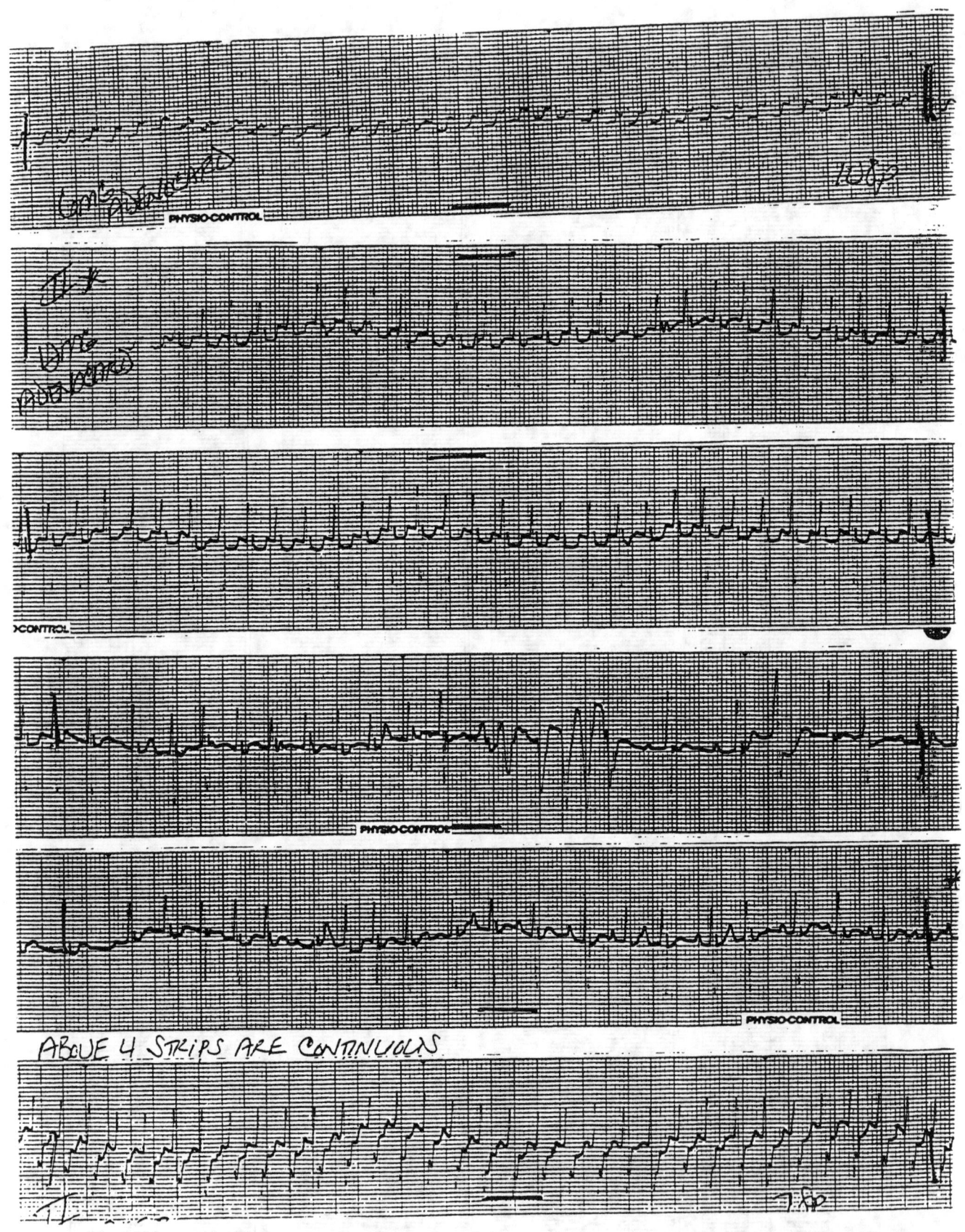

ABOVE 4 STRIPS ARE CONTINUOUS

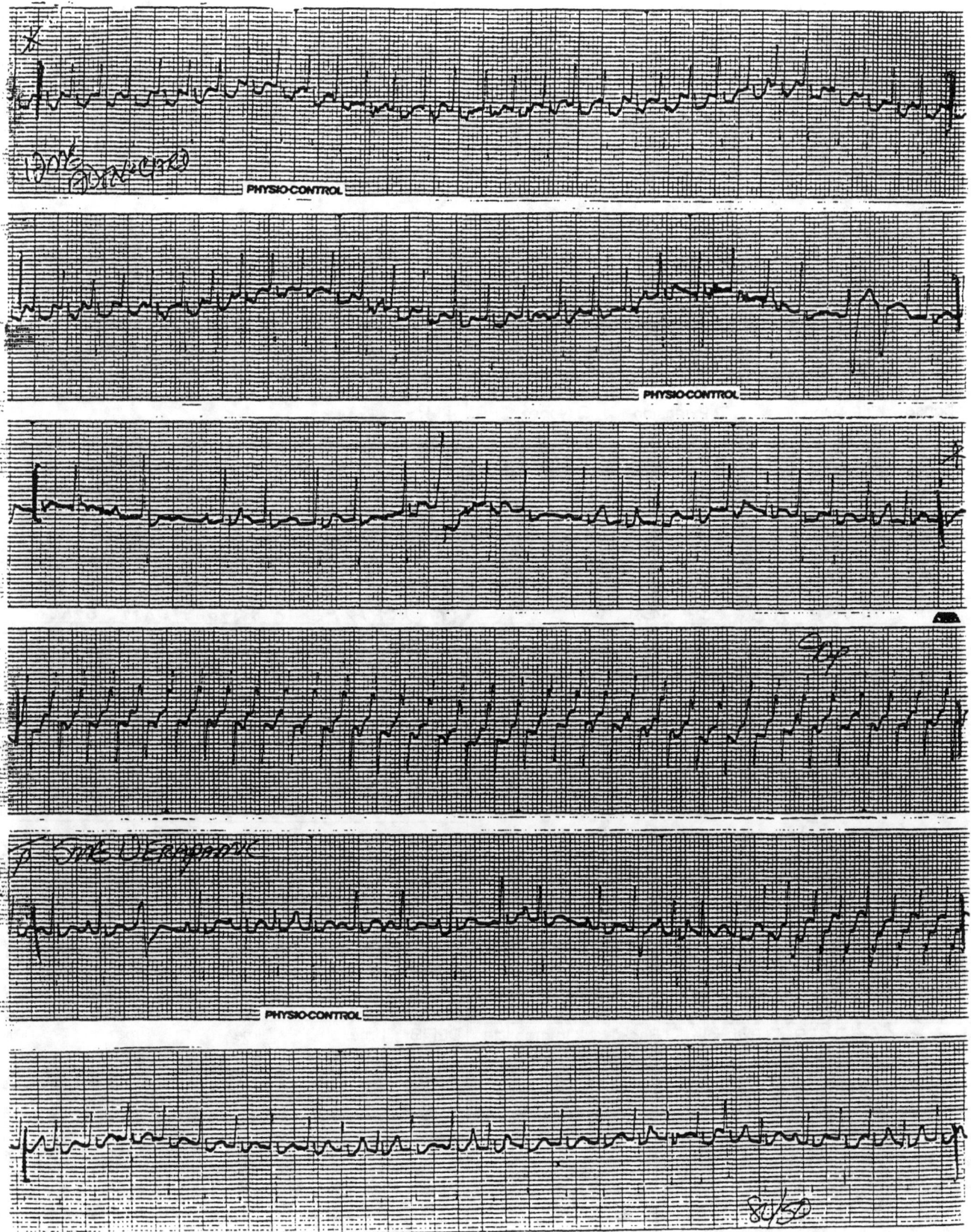

E.M.S. TRAINING PROGRAM
PATIENT CARE REPORT FORM

© 1992 Kennedy Associate

Patient Name: Margaret Eaton	Trip #: 039 Date: 30 Sept. 1992
Address: 35 White St.	M.R.#: Day: Wednesday
Boston MA	Dispatch To: For: ? Respiratory
DOB: 18 April 1895 Tel. #:	35 White St. 6th floor #601
Next of Kin:	Dispatch Time: 0022 Arrival Time: 0028
Address:	To Hospital: 0013 At Hospital: 0015
	Location at Dispatch: Cross + Main Sts.
Relationship: Tel. #:	Billing Information (circle):
Transported to: Trauma Gen Hosp Transport Priority: 1	(Medicare) Medicaid BC/BS
Miles from: 008.4 To: 011.2	Indust. Acc. Self Other
❏ No Transport	Subscriber: Patient
REASON:	
	Policy #: 020 406120 A

Physical Exam

Eye Opening: ☒ Spontaneous ❏ To Pain ❏ To Voice ❏ None

Verbal Response: ☒ Oriented ❏ Confused ❏ Inappropriate ❏ Incomprehensible ❏ None

Motor Response: ☒ Obedience ❏ Purposeful ❏ Withdrawal ❏ Flexion ❏ Extension ❏ None

Skin Condition: ❏ Normal ❏ Cool ❏ Hot ❏ Pale ❏ Flushed ❏ Cyanotic ☒ Diaphoretic (mildly)

Vital Signs

❏ Unable to Obtain   ❏ Not attempted
REASON:

Time	BP	Pulse	Resp. Rate/Effort
	See Narrative		

Allergies: ☒ None / ❏ Unknown

Current Medications: See narrative / ❏ None / ❏ Unknown

Brought with Pt.? ❏ Yes ❏ No

Suspected Diagnosis: ❏ Chronic ☒ Acute
❏ Major Trauma ❏ Acute Medical ❏ Cardiac Arrest ❏ Shock
❏ Minor Trauma ❏ Minor Medical ☒ Cardiac Disorder ❏ ETOH
❏ Soft Tissue Injury ❏ Burns ❏ Ortho ❏ OD/Poison
❏ Neuro ❏ Seizure ❏ Psych ❏ OB/GYN ❏ Neonate

Chief Complaint/History/Changes in Patient Status

S.O.B.

97 yo f found supine in bed in 6th floor apt.
(HPI) Pt is c/o 2° hx of SOB, onset while preparing for bed. (1) 0.15 mg NTG 1° ago c̄ relief now also vomiting. c/o bilat lower abd pain + dizziness

(PE) A/ox3 Skin warm, dry c̄ Normal color, neck veins mildly distended. Trach midline. BBS ⊖ c̄ rales throughout. ⊕ access. musc. use + IC retractions - abd soft, nontender. moderate pedal edema. BP (seated) 180/100 EKG: AF @ 130-140/min Some unifocal ectopy RR 48

(PMH) CHF/PE in distant past. other hx is unclear. meds: 0.15 NTG Tabs 0.125 Halcion NKA

(TX) O2 → IV → NTG → NTG/Lasix BP 190/100. Spontaneous conversion to SR @ 120-130/min c̄ frequent PAC's → NTG/MS → BP 180/100 RR 36 No other △. mildly Diaphoretic at arrival at Hospital

Advanced Life Support

Time	Medication	Rate/Dose	Route
0049	D5W	KVO	22g ®ha
0052	NTG	0.4 mg	SL Spray
0054	NTG	0.4 mg	SL Spray
0059	Lasix	60 mg	IV
0100	NTG	0.4 mg	SL Spray
0102	MS	2 mg	IV
0113	NTG	0.4 mg	SL Spray

Total Fluid Infused: mls

Emergency Care: ❏ CPR ❏ Extricate ❏ Back/Neck Immobilize
❏ Bleed Control ❏ Bandage ❏ Splint ❏ Heat/Cold Applied
☒ O2 Administration: 15 liters/minute via NRB
Airway: ❏ Cleared ❏ Oral ❏ Nasal Size: ___ ❏ Suction
Intubate: ❏ Endotracheal ❏ Nasotracheal Size: _____
Assist Ventilation: Rate: ___ Method: ___
☒ ECG Monitor ☒ Rhythm Strip Attached
Transport Position: Fowlers

DEFIB: Time:	Time:	Time:	Time:
Joules:	Joules:	Joules:	Joules:

Medical Control: ❏ Direct ☒ C-MED Channel 5
MD# 33   Hospital _____
Hospital Notified Enroute: ☒ Yes ❏ No
☒ C-MED ❏ Dispatcher

Other Response Units/Agencies:

Unit # P9   EMT/Paramedic Signatures: _Cathleen Diaz_ # 196   _Hugh Morton_ # 165   #

Trip # 039

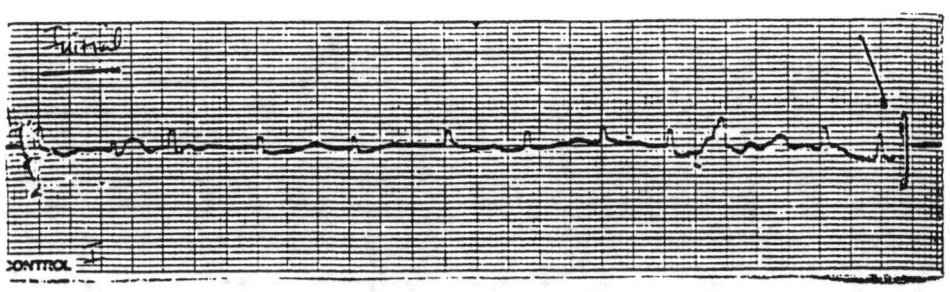

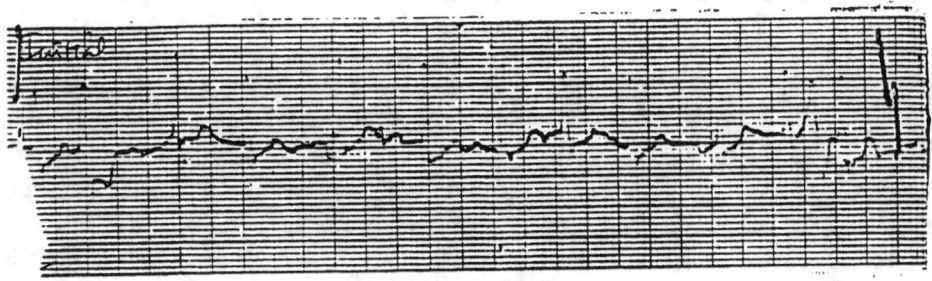

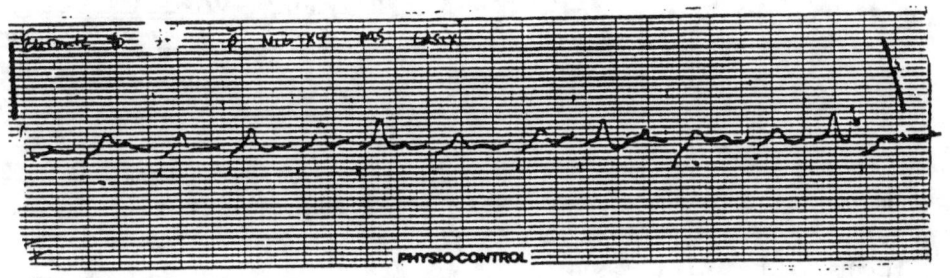

E.M.S. TRAINING PROGRAM
PATIENT CARE REPORT FORM

© 1992 Kennedy Associates

Patient Name: Dorothy Evans	Trip #: 040 Date: 9-30-92
Address: 109 Riverway avenue	M.R.#: Day: Wed.
Boston MA	Dispatch To: For: S.O.B. + cardiac
DOB: 10-15-16 Tel. #: 555-6259	109 Riverway Ave
Next of Kin: Michael Evans	Dispatch Time: 1314 Arrival Time: 1321
Address: S/A	To Hospital: 1331 At Hospital: 1342
	Location at Dispatch: Station 2
Relationship: Husband Tel. #: Same	Billing Information (circle):
Transported to: Community Hosp Transport Priority: 1	(Medicare) Medicaid BC/BS
Miles from: 452.6 To: 460.1	Indust. Acc. Self Other
❑ No Transport	Subscriber:
REASON:	
	Policy #: 105 60 2160 B

Physical Exam

Eye Opening	❑ Spontaneous ☒ To Voice	❑ To Pain ❑ None
Verbal Response	☒ Oriented ❑ Inappropriate	❑ Confused ❑ Incomprehensible ❑ None
Motor Response	☒ Obedience ❑ Flexion	❑ Purposeful ❑ Extension ❑ Withdrawal ❑ None
Skin Condition	❑ Normal ❑ Cool ❑ Hot ☒ Pale ❑ Flushed ❑ Cyanotic ☒ Diaphoretic	

Vital Signs

❑ Unable to Obtain   ❑ Not attempted
REASON:

Time	BP	Pulse	Resp. Rate/Effort
1340 (EMT)	110/70	150	40 shallow/labored
1328	130/P	150	40 shallow/labored
1341	134/P	150	40 shallow/labored

Allergies: ❑ None ☒ Unknown

Current Medications: *See note*   ❑ None ❑ Unknown

Brought with Pt.? ❑ Yes ☒ No

Suspected Diagnosis: ❑ Chronic ☒ Acute
❑ Major Trauma ☒ Acute Medical ❑ Cardiac Arrest ❑ Shock
❑ Minor Trauma ❑ Minor Medical ☒ Cardiac Disorder ❑ ETOH
❑ Soft Tissue Injury ❑ Burns ❑ Ortho ❑ OD/Poison
❑ Neuro ❑ Seizure ❑ Psych ❑ OB/GYN ❑ Neonate

Emergency Care: ❑ CPR ☒ Extricate ❑ Back/Neck Immobilize
❑ Bleed Control ❑ Bandage ❑ Splint ❑ Heat/Cold Applied
☒ O₂ Administration: 12 liters/minute via Non-Rebreather
Airway: ❑ Cleared ❑ Oral ❑ Nasal Size: ___ ❑ Suction
Intubate: ❑ Endotracheal ❑ Nasotracheal Size: ___
Assist Ventilation: Rate: ___ Method: ___
☒ ECG Monitor ☒ Rhythm Strip Attached
Transport Position: Upright on stretcher

Unit #: P2   EMT/Paramedic Signatures: Jeff Rawson # 148 Dean Raven # 135   #

Chief Complaint/History/Changes in Patient Status

75yo ♀ S.O.B.

(HPI) acute onset aprox. 1245 to 1300 HRS today presents to BLS as S.O.B. + Tachycardic. Presents to ALS in BLS ambulance

(PMH) cardio-respiratory including MI during the past few weeks; diabetes

(MEDS) Procardia; TNG 1/150; captopril; Isordil Var TID; Digoxin 0.125mg; albuterol; atrovent; colace; Lasix 20mg; Prednisone, Zantac; multivits; Immuran; unknown if any allergies

(PE) conscious, oriented, severe dyspnea speaks single word answers only to questions. Skin pale + diaphor. B.S. Rhonci + wheeze Inspiratory + Expiratory all fiel. note retraction of accessory muscles. ECG is sinus Tachycardia @ 150/min RR 40 labored/shallow BP 130/p abd soft/nontender, moves arms+legs spontaneously

(Rx) ↑Fi O₂ mask, change to proventil treatment establish IV D5W KVO, draw bloods, admin Nitrospray D-Ye x2, and Lasix 40mg IVP, slight change to speaking in clipped phrases. Vital signs S.A. Consider E.T. Tube.

Advanced Life Support

Time	Medication	Rate/Dose	Route
1330	Proventil	0.5 in 2.5 NS	Inhalation
1330	D5W	KVO	18gauge © AC
1335	TNG	0.4mg x 2	SL Spray
1335	Lasix	40mg	IVP

Total Fluid Infused: <50 mls

DEFIB: Time:	Time:	Time:	Time:
Joules:	Joules:	Joules:	Joules:

Medical Control: ❑ Direct ❑ C-MED Channel 3
MD#___   Hospital ___
Hospital Notified Enroute: ☒ Yes ❑ No
☒ C-MED ❑ Dispatcher

Other Response Units/Agencies:

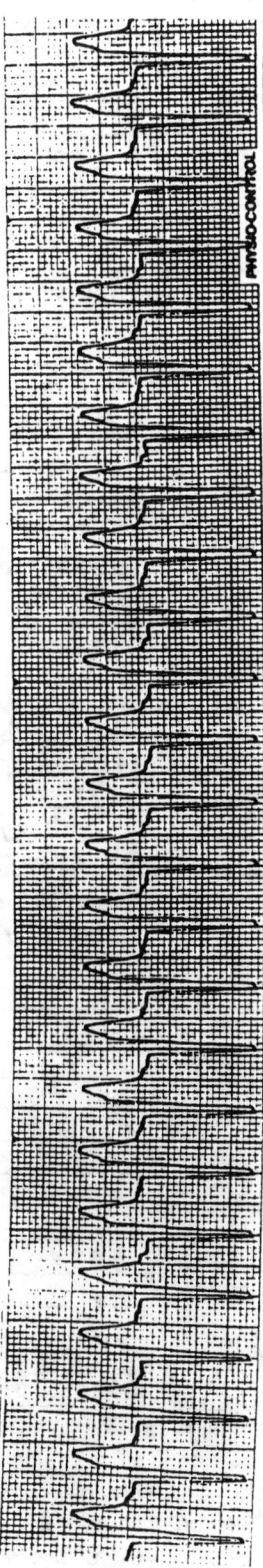

Trip #040

E.M.S. TRAINING PROGRAM
PATIENT CARE REPORT FORM

© 1992 Kennedy Associate

Patient Name: *Marta Hernandez*	Trip #: *041* Date: *09/30/92*
Address: *98 Broadlawn Way*	M.R.#: *002 60 51 6* Day: *Wed*
Boston MA	Dispatch To: For: *Cardiac*
DOB: *06/15/78* Tel. #: *555-5609*	*98 Broadlawn Wy*
Next of Kin: *Pedro Hernandez*	Dispatch Time: *1656* Arrival Time: *1705*
Address: *S/A*	To Hospital: *1750* At Hospital: *1805*

Location at Dispatch:

Relationship: *Father*   Tel. #: *Same*

Billing Information (circle):

Transported to: *TGH*   Transport Priority:

Miles from: To:

Medicare   Medicaid   BC/BS

Indust. Acc.   Self   Other

❏ No Transport
REASON:

Subscriber:

Info not Available

Policy #:

Physical Exam

Eye Opening	☒ Spontaneous ❏ To Pain	❏ To Voice ❏ None
Verbal Response	☒ Oriented ❏ Confused	❏ Inappropriate ❏ Incomprehensible ❏ None
Motor Response	☒ Obedience ❏ Purposeful ❏ Withdrawal	❏ Flexion ❏ Extension ❏ None
Skin Condition	❏ Normal ☒ Cool ❏ Hot ❏ Pale	❏ Flushed ❏ Cyanotic ❏ Diaphoretic

Vital Signs

❏ Unable to Obtain   ❏ Not attempted
REASON:

Time	BP	Pulse	Resp. Rate/Effort
1712	76/P	190	24
1730	76/P	190	24
1800	102/70	90	20

Allergies: ☒ None   ❏ Unknown

Current Medications: ❏ None   ❏ Unknown

Brought with Pt.? ❏ Yes ❏ No

Suspected Diagnosis: ❏ Chronic ☒ Acute
❏ Major Trauma ❏ Acute Medical ❏ Cardiac Arrest ❏ Shock
❏ Minor Trauma ❏ Minor Medical ☒ Cardiac Disorder ❏ ETOH
❏ Soft Tissue Injury ❏ Burns ❏ Ortho ❏ OD/Poison
❏ Neuro ❏ Seizure ❏ Psych ❏ OB/GYN ❏ Neonate

Emergency Care: ❏ CPR ❏ Extricate ❏ Back/Neck Immobilize
❏ Bleed Control ❏ Bandage ❏ Splint ❏ Heat/Cold Applied
☒ O₂ Administration: *10* liters/minute via *N/R*
Airway: ❏ Cleared ❏ Oral ❏ Nasal Size: _____ ❏ Suction
Intubate: ❏ Endotracheal ❏ Nasotracheal Size: _____
Assist Ventilation: Rate: _____ Method: _____
❏ ECG Monitor ❏ Rhythm Strip Attached
Transport Position: *Supine*

Chief Complaint/History/Changes in Patient Status

14 y/o Spanish speaking ♀ who, per family, has had chest pain, palpitations + nausea x 3 hours c̄ hx P.A.T.
PE: CA+o x3 Skin cool + dry c̄ good color breath sounds c = Bilat. ECG SVT @ 190
PMH: PAT
MEDS: Atenolol
NKA
TX: placed on high flow O₂ I.V. NS started
1724: Adenosine 6mg IV s̄ Δ
1728: Adenosine 12mg IV + 500cc Bolus NS s̄ Δ
1734 Adenosine 12mg IV Pt. broke to a sinus Rhythm @ 90 c̄ ? WPW
Pt. BP ↑ TX 102/70 + now s̄ complaint
Vagal maneuvers attempted prior to 1st 12mg of Adenosine s̄ Δ

Advanced Life Support

Time	/ Medication /	Rate/Dose /	Route
1722	NS 1000mL	500cc Bolus	#18 (R) fossa
1724	Adenosine	6mg	IV
1728	Adenosine	12mg	IV
1734	Adenosine	12mg	IV
/	/	/	
/	/	/	
/	/	/	

Total Fluid Infused: *500* mls

DEFIB: Time:	Time:	Time:	Time:
Joules:	Joules:	Joules:	Joules:

Medical Control: ❏ Direct ☒ C-MED Channel *8*
MD# *48*   Hospital _____
Hospital Notified Enroute: ☒ Yes ❏ No
☒ C-MED ❏ Dispatcher

Other Response Units/Agencies:

Unit # *P1*   EMT/Paramedic Signatures:
John Middleton # *152*   *Harry James* # *153*   #

Trip #041 page 1 of 2

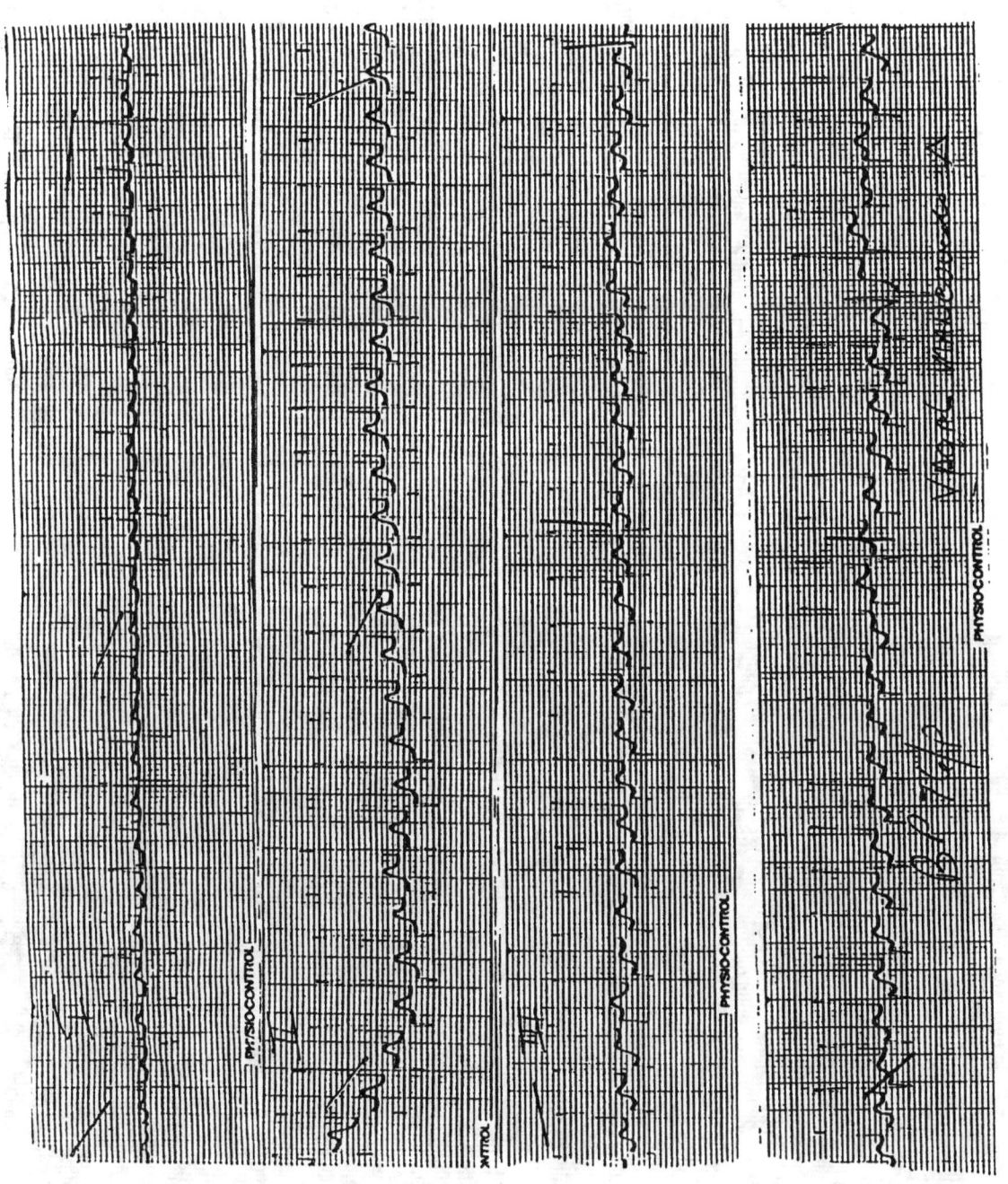

Trip #041 page 2 of 2

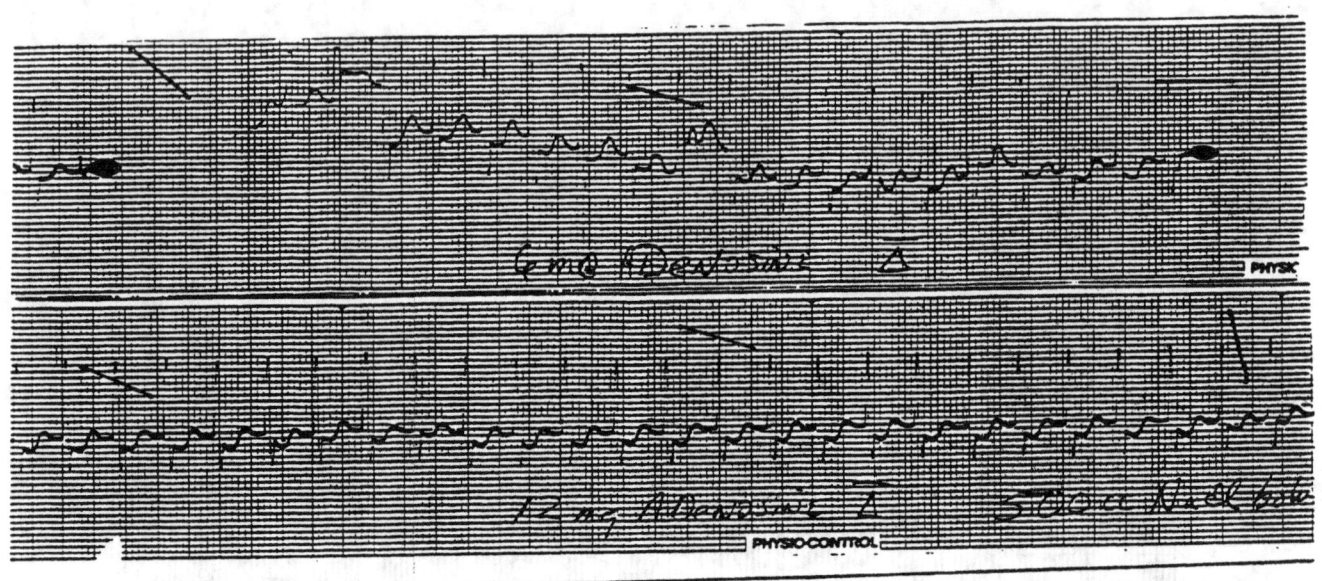

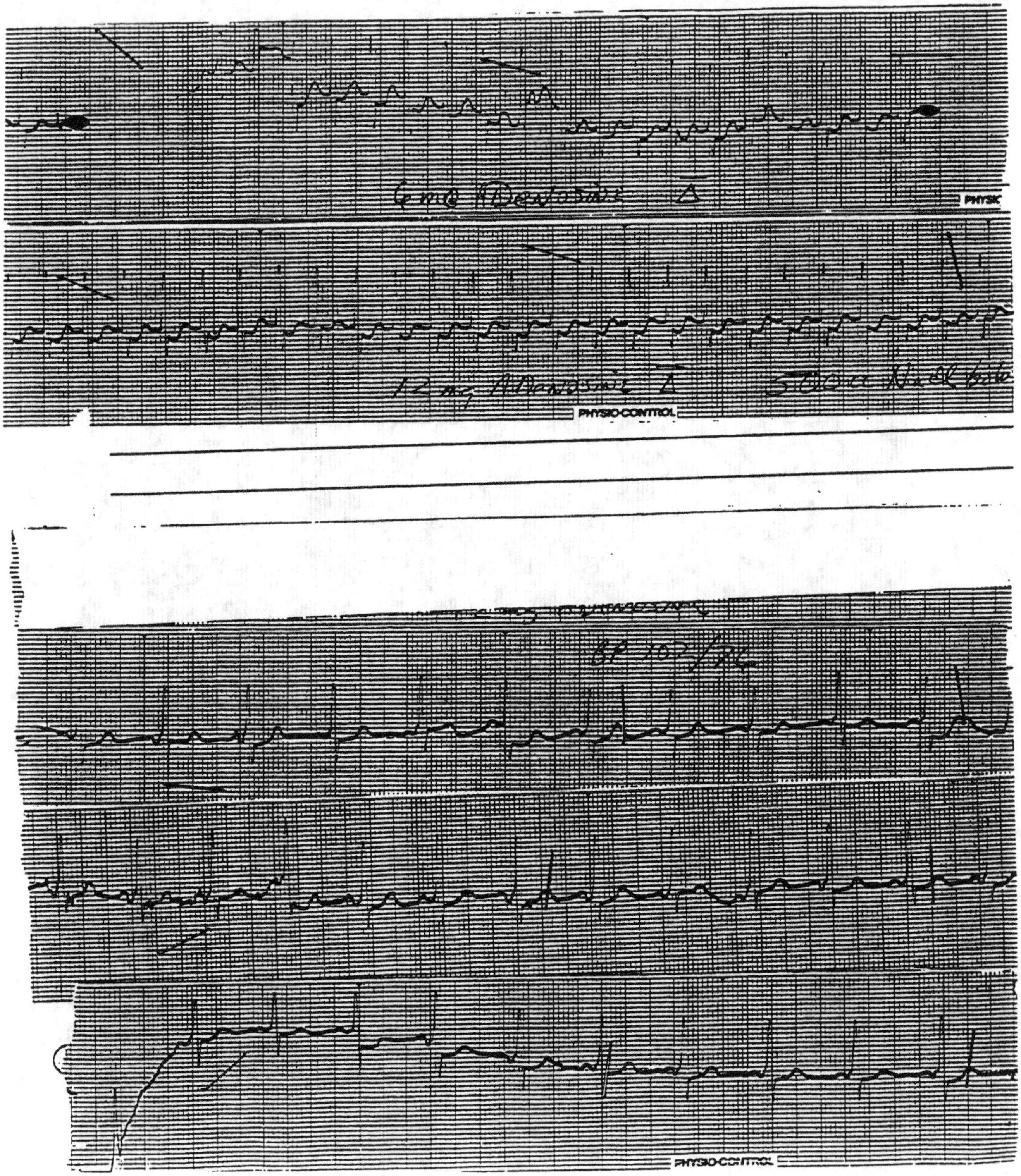

Notes

© 1992 Kennedy Associate

E.M.S. TRAINING PROGRAM
PATIENT CARE REPORT FORM

Patient Name: Georgia Fuller	Trip #: 042 / Date: 09/30/92
Address: 16 Walden ST	M.R.#: / Day: Wed
Boston MA	Dispatch To: / For: Heart Problem
DOB: 12/24/16 Tel. #: 555-4389	16 Walden ST
Next of Kin: Samuel Hewitt	Dispatch Time: / Arrival Time:
Address: 18 Walden ST	To Hospital: / At Hospital:
Boston MA	Location at Dispatch:
Relationship: Brother Tel. #: 555-8718	Billing Information (circle):
Transported to: Community Hosp Transport Priority: 1	Medicare Medicaid BC/BS
Miles from: To:	Indust. Acc. Self Other
❏ No Transport	Subscriber:
REASON:	
	Policy #:

Physical Exam

Eye Opening: ☒ Spontaneous ❏ To Pain ❏ To Voice ❏ None

Verbal Response: ☒ Oriented ❏ Confused ❏ Inappropriate ❏ Incomprehensible ❏ None

Motor Response: ☒ Obedience ❏ Purposeful ❏ Withdrawal ❏ Flexion ❏ Extension ❏ None

Skin Condition: ☒ Normal ❏ Cool ❏ Hot ❏ Pale ❏ Flushed ❏ Cyanotic ❏ Diaphoretic

Vital Signs

❏ Unable to Obtain   ❏ Not attempted
REASON:

Time	BP	Pulse	Resp. Rate/Effort
1955	200/120	70	20
2005	180/P	60	20
2020	170/100	60	20

Allergies: ❏ None ☒ Unknown

Current Medications: ❏ None ❏ Unknown

Brought with Pt.? ❏ Yes ☒ No

Suspected Diagnosis: ❏ Chronic ❏ Acute
❏ Major Trauma ❏ Acute Medical ❏ Cardiac Arrest ❏ Shock
❏ Minor Trauma ❏ Minor Medical ☒ Cardiac Disorder ❏ ETOH
❏ Soft Tissue Injury ❏ Burns ❏ Ortho ❏ OD/Poison
❏ Neuro ❏ Seizure ❏ Psych ❏ OB/GYN ❏ Neonate

Chief Complaint/History/Changes in Patient Status

75 y/o ♀ at home in bed c/o L sided chest non Radiating unrelieved by TNG at home c similar episode this afternoon. Pt has pmh of angina, HTN.

Pt con A+O x3 4mm Pupils React warm dry skin c good color Norm cap refill ⊖ JVD Lungs clear =
EKG - NSR 60-70 s ectopy Denies nausea vomiting s Pedal Edema

Pt treated c 4L nasal O₂ - IV D5W KVO
1 SL TNG 1/150 c some improvement
p̄ 5 minutes given another SL TNG 1/150
c more improvement however still c/o
Pain arrival at hosp

Advanced Life Support

Time	/	Medication	/	Rate/Dose	/	Route
2000	/	D5W	/	KVO	/	120° (L) hand
2005	/	TNG	/	0.4 mg	/	SL
2020	/	TNG	/	0.4 mg	/	SL
	/		/		/	
	/		/		/	
	/		/		/	
	/		/		/	

Total Fluid Infused: 10 mls

Emergency Care: ❏ CPR ❏ Extricate ❏ Back/Neck Immobilize
❏ Bleed Control ❏ Bandage ❏ Splint ❏ Heat/Cold Applied
☒ O₂ Administration: 4 liters/minute via Nasal
Airway: ❏ Cleared ❏ Oral ❏ Nasal Size: _____ ❏ Suction
Intubate: ❏ Endotracheal ❏ Nasotracheal Size: _____
Assist Ventilation: Rate: _____ Method: _____
☒ ECG Monitor ☒ Rhythm Strip Attached
Transport Position: Semi Fowler

DEFIB: Time:	Time:	Time:	Time:
Joules:	Joules:	Joules:	Joules:

Medical Control: ❏ Direct ☒ C-MED Channel _____
MD# _____ Hospital _____
Hospital Notified Enroute: ☒ Yes ❏ No
☒ C-MED ❏ Dispatcher

Other Response Units/Agencies:

Unit #: P16   EMT/Paramedic Signatures:
Tracy Peters # 191   # _____   # _____

Trip #042

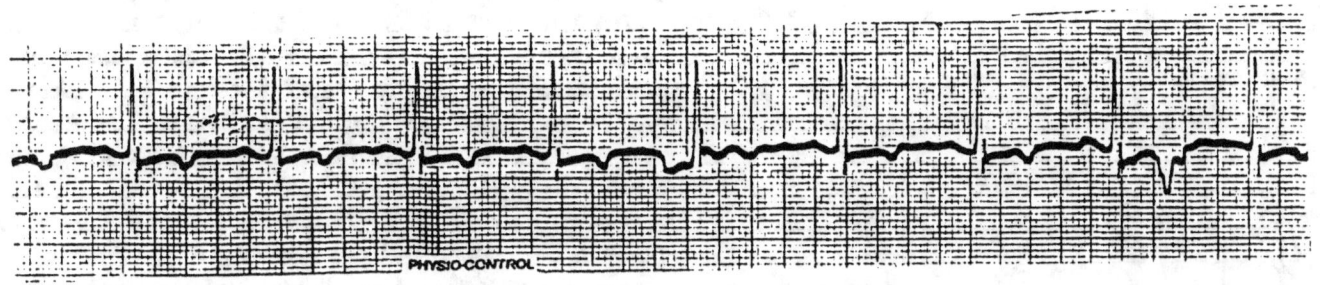

E.M.S. TRAINING PROGRAM
PATIENT CARE REPORT FORM

© 1992 Kennedy Associates

Patient Name: John Noonan	Trip #: 043 / Date: 09/30/92
Address: 48 5th Avenue	M.R.#: / Day: Wednesday
Newton MA	Dispatch To: For: MVA
DOB: 01-30-66 Tel. #: 555-4154	1800 Washington Blvd
Next of Kin: Kenneth Noonan	Dispatch Time: 0204 Arrival Time: 0210
Address: 12 Barrows St	To Hospital: 0228 At Hospital: 0245
Waltham MA	Location at Dispatch: ~~Station~~ Quarters
Relationship: Father Tel. #: 555-6682	Billing Information (circle):
Transported to: T.G.H. Transport Priority: 1	Medicare Medicaid BC/BS
Miles from: To:	Indust. Acc. Self Other
❏ No Transport REASON:	Subscriber:
	Policy #:

Physical Exam

Eye Opening	☒ Spontaneous ❏ To Pain	
	❏ To Voice ❏ None	
Verbal Response	☒ Oriented ❏ Confused	
	❏ Inappropriate ❏ Incomprehensible ❏ None	
Motor Response	☒ Obedience ❏ Purposeful ❏ Withdrawal	
	❏ Flexion ❏ Extension ❏ None	
Skin Condition	☒ Normal ❏ Cool ❏ Hot ❏ Pale	
	❏ Flushed ❏ Cyanotic ❏ Diaphoretic	

Vital Signs

❏ Unable to Obtain   ❏ Not attempted
REASON:

Time	BP	Pulse	Resp. Rate/Effort
0214	146/P	92	20
0226	110/P	88	20
0233	130/P	88	20
0241	136/P	80	20

Allergies: ❏ None   ☒ Unknown

Current Medications: ❏ None   ☒ Unknown

Brought with Pt.?   ❏ Yes   ❏ No

Suspected Diagnosis: ❏ Chronic ☒ Acute
☒ Major Trauma ❏ Acute Medical ❏ Cardiac Arrest ❏ Shock
❏ Minor Trauma ❏ Minor Medical ❏ Cardiac Disorder ❏ ETOH
❏ Soft Tissue Injury ❏ Burns ❏ Ortho ❏ OD/Poison
❏ Neuro ❏ Seizure ❏ Psych ❏ OB/GYN ❏ Neonate

Emergency Care: ❏ CPR ❏ Extricate ❏ Back/Neck Immobilize
☒ Bleed Control ☒ Bandage ☒ Splint ❏ Heat/Cold Applied
☒ O₂ Administration: 15 liters/minute via NRB
Airway: ❏ Cleared ❏ Oral ❏ Nasal Size: _____ ❏ Suction
Intubate: ❏ Endotracheal ❏ Nasotracheal Size: _____
Assist Ventilation: Rate: _____ Method: _____
☒ ECG Monitor ❏ Rhythm Strip Attached
Transport Position:

Chief Complaint/History/Changes in Patient Status

Chief Complaint - Trauma to ® hand S/P MVA
H) PT Passenger (? used restraint) in open jeep
that rolled over landing on roof area PT states
he did not lose L.O.C. and was removed from his seat
by bystanders @ scene PT admits to 9 alcoholic beverages
hx meds allergies unknown
4) CAOx3 26♀ supine on pavement c̄ ® hand up
trying to control bleeding. Pt wt aprox 80 kg
HEENT ⊖ obvious trauma. PERLA facial bones intact
⊖ teeth noted missing ⊖ JVD Trachea midline ⊖ Subcutaneous
emphysema noted. C-spine ⊖ chest intact c̄ symmetrical
movement c̄ good tidal volume. is clear ⊕ bilat. ⊖ bruising or
lacerations noted abd soft nontender. ⊖ bruising and
lacerations noted Pelvis intact. lower extremities unremarkable
PT able to move extremities c̄ good sensation. upper
extremities: LUE unremarkable RUE massive avulsion
to dorsal aspect from wrist distally c̄ bone + tendon visible
Deformity noted. PT has sensation in fingertips to ® hand
Remainder exam ⊖ V/S as noted ECG NSR @ 88 ⊖ ectopy
EBL 250-500 cc

Advanced Life Support

Time	Medication	Rate/Dose	Route
Rx) c-spine immobilize IHf flow O₂ IV LR ⊕ Arm
IV NS ® Arm AC DSD to wound splint, Bleeding
Control
1) Trauma Center-Exam repeated en route several times
s̄ Δ Transported c̄ incident
0224	NS	KVO	146A ® AC
0335	LR	KVO	146A ⓛ AC

Total Fluid Infused: 250 mls

DEFIB:	Time:	Time:	Time:	Time:
	Joules:	Joules:	Joules:	Joules:

Medical Control: ❏ Direct ❏ C-MED Channel _____
MD# _____ Hospital _____
Hospital Notified Enroute: ❏ Yes ❏ No
❏ C-MED ❏ Dispatcher

Other Response Units/Agencies:
Police + Fire

| Unit # P7 | EMT/Paramedic Signatures: Thomas Larkin # 130   Kevin Harden # 128   # |

E.M.S. TRAINING PROGRAM
PATIENT CARE REPORT FORM

© 1992 Kennedy Associates

Patient Name: Bing Ho	Trip #: 044 — Date: 09/30/92
Address: 94 Wrentham Ter.	M.R.#: — Day: Wednesday
Boston MA	Dispatch To: / For: Unconscious
DOB: 1924 Tel. #:	14 Oak St
Next of Kin:	Dispatch Time: 1135 — Arrival Time: 1148
Address:	To Hospital: 1205 — At Hospital: 1215
	Location at Dispatch:
Relationship: — Tel. #:	Billing Information (circle):
Transported to: C.H. — Transport Priority:	Medicare Medicaid BC/BS
Miles from: — To:	(Indust. Acc.) Self Other
☐ No Transport	Subscriber:
REASON:	Policy #:

Physical Exam

Eye Opening	☒ Spontaneous ☐ To Pain
	☐ To Voice ☐ None
Verbal Response	☒ Oriented ☐ Confused
	☐ Inappropriate ☐ Incomprehensible ☐ None
Motor Response	☒ Obedience ☐ Purposeful ☐ Withdrawal
	☐ Flexion ☐ Extension ☐ None
Skin Condition	☐ Normal ☐ Cool ☒ Hot ☐ Pale
	☐ Flushed ☐ Cyanotic ☐ Diaphoretic

Vital Signs

☐ Unable to Obtain   ☐ Not attempted
REASON:

Time	BP	Pulse	Resp. Rate/Effort
1150	160/92	88	14 mild-labored
1205	160/58	84	12 mild labored

Allergies: ☒ None
                                              ☐ Unknown

Current Medications: ☒ None
                                              ☐ Unknown

Brought with Pt.?   ☐ Yes   ☐ No

Suspected Diagnosis: ☐ Chronic ☒ Acute
☐ Major Trauma ☐ Acute Medical ☐ Cardiac Arrest ☐ Shock
☐ Minor Trauma ☐ Minor Medical ☐ Cardiac Disorder ☐ ETOH
☐ Soft Tissue Injury ☒ Burns ☐ Ortho ☐ OD/Poison
☐ Neuro ☐ Seizure ☐ Psych ☐ OB/GYN ☐ Neonate

Chief Complaint/History/Changes in Patient Status

BLS arrived to find a conscious, non-English speaking 68 y/o ♂ lying on ground after working w/ a chemical that is a hydrocarbon resin that flashed over exploding in his face. Pt. complains of inability to see, has sensation above his face and neck and a warm sensation when he breathes. ALS arrived found BLS flushing pt's eyes and skin w/ sterile water. Pt complaints as noted. PE skin hot and dry w/ no visible burn marks w/ redness and swelling around both eyes, eyebrows singed, nose hair gone. No signs of burns or edema in oropharynx. Trachea midline. Good BS = + clear w/ good tidal volume, no burn marks on hands. Pt denies PMH, meds or allergies. MD contacted ordered IV LR KVO established Ⓛ forearm 16ga 1½" first attempt and monitor enroute Pt eyes + face constantly flushed w/ NS IV flush and complained only of burning sensation, denied S.O.B. w/ no change in Pt status or condition noted

Advanced Life Support

Time	/	Medication	/	Rate/Dose	/	Route
1157	/	L.R.	/	KVO	/	16ga 1½ Ⓛ for
	/		/		/	
	/		/		/	
	/		/		/	
	/		/		/	
	/		/		/	
	/		/		/	
	/		/		/	

Total Fluid Infused: _____ mls

Emergency Care: ☐ CPR ☐ Extricate ☐ Back/Neck Immobilize
☐ Bleed Control ☐ Bandage ☐ Splint ☐ Heat/Cold Applied
☒ O₂ Administration: 10 liters/minute via NRB
Airway: ☐ Cleared ☐ Oral ☐ Nasal Size: ___ ☐ Suction
Intubate: ☐ Endotracheal ☐ Nasotracheal Size: ___
Assist Ventilation: Rate: ___ Method: ___
☐ ECG Monitor ☐ Rhythm Strip Attached
Transport Position: Supine

DEFIB:	Time:	Time:	Time:	Time:
	Joules:	Joules:	Joules:	Joules:

Medical Control: ☐ Direct ☒ C-MED Channel 8
MD# 61   Hospital _____
Hospital Notified Enroute: ☒ Yes   ☐ No
                             ☒ C-MED   ☐ Dispatcher

Other Response Units/Agencies:
Fire Dept

Unit # P13   EMT/Paramedic Signatures:
Von Paige   # 177   T-G.   # 186   _____ #_____

E.M.S. TRAINING PROGRAM
PATIENT CARE REPORT FORM

© 1992 Kennedy Associates

Patient Name: Jill Harrison	Trip #: 045 Date: 9-30-1992
Address: 1429 Parkway Blvd	M.R.#: Day: Wed.
Boston MA	Dispatch To: For: cardiac
DOB: 3-22-84 Tel. #:	Community Health Clinic
Next of Kin: Susan Harrison	Dispatch Time: 1533 Arrival Time: 1539
Address: 1429 Parkway Blvd	To Hospital: 1652 At Hospital: 1700
Boston MA	Location at Dispatch: Quarters
Relationship: Mother Tel. #: 555-3203	Billing Information (circle):
Transported to: Comm. Hosp Transport Priority: 1	Medicare Medicaid (BC/BS)
Miles from: To:	Indust. Acc. Self Other
❑ No Transport	Subscriber: Mother
REASON:	Policy #: 000 43 68579

Physical Exam

Eye Opening: ☒ Spontaneous ❑ To Pain ❑ To Voice ❑ None

Verbal Response: ☒ Oriented ❑ Confused ❑ Inappropriate ❑ Incomprehensible ❑ None

Motor Response: ☒ Obedience ❑ Purposeful ❑ Withdrawal ❑ Flexion ❑ Extension ❑ None

Skin Condition: ☒ Normal ❑ Cool ❑ Hot ❑ Pale ❑ Flushed ❑ Cyanotic ❑ Diaphoretic

Vital Signs

❑ Unable to Obtain   ❑ Not attempted
REASON:

Time	BP	Pulse	Resp. Rate/Effort
1550	148/84	150	20
1630	150/100	150	20
1650	160/88	110	18

Allergies: ☒ None ❑ Unknown

Current Medications: ❑ None ❑ Unknown

See comments

Brought with Pt.? ❑ Yes ❑ No

Suspected Diagnosis: ❑ Chronic ❑ Acute
❑ Major Trauma ❑ Acute Medical ❑ Cardiac Arrest ❑ Shock
❑ Minor Trauma ❑ Minor Medical ❑ Cardiac Disorder ❑ ETOH
❑ Soft Tissue Injury ❑ Burns ❑ Ortho ❑ OD/Poison
❑ Neuro ❑ Seizure ❑ Psych ❑ OB/GYN ❑ Neonate

Emergency Care: ❑ CPR ❑ Extricate ❑ Back/Neck Immobilize
❑ Bleed Control ❑ Bandage ❑ Splint ❑ Heat/Cold Applied
☒ O₂ Administration: 4 liters/minute via NASAL
Airway: ❑ Cleared ❑ Oral ❑ Nasal Size: ____ ❑ Suction
Intubate: ❑ Endotracheal ❑ Nasotracheal Size: _____
Assist Ventilation: Rate: _____ Method: _____
☒ ECG Monitor ☒ Rhythm Strip Attached
Transport Position: Semi-Fowler

Unit # P10

Chief Complaint/History/Changes in Patient Status

8 yo ♀ seen at Community Health Clinic for new onset of bilateral pitting edema and intermittent SSCP. 12 lead ECG was done & was found to be in an SVT at 150 ST in leads 2, 3, V₂-V₆ & AVF. Upon our arrival pt. presents CAOx3 good color, warm & dry Ø JVD BS clear & = bilat. 3+ bilat pitting pedal edema. ECG SVT at 150 ST ↓ in leads II + III. PMH SVT. meds: dig, Calan, quinidine NKA. Pt. placed on 4 lpm nasal O₂. Initially pt. refusing any treatment however eventually consented. Rec'd an IV NaCl KVO adm 6mg Adenocard IV broke SVT to sinus GT 100 ST ↓ in lead II. Rec'd .4mg SL NTG enroute to hospital SL

Advanced Life Support

Time	/ Medication /	Rate/Dose	/ Route
1630	NaCl	KVO	@ AC #18g
1635	Adenocard	6mg	IVP
1645	NTG	.4mg	SL
/	/	/	
/	/	/	
/	/	/	
/	/	/	

Total Fluid Infused: ____ mls

DEFIB: Time: Time: Time: Time:
Joules: Joules: Joules: Joules:

Medical Control: ❑ Direct ❑ C-MED Channel _____
MD# 45   Hospital _____
Hospital Notified Enroute: ❑ Yes ❑ No
❑ C-MED ❑ Dispatcher

Other Response Units/Agencies:

EMT/Paramedic Signatures: David Seward # 188   Jan Teano # 199   # ____

Trip #045 page 1 of 2

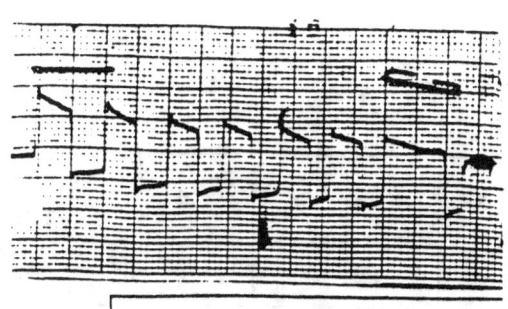

PRE-HOSPITAL ECG   lead I   PAGE 1 OF 2

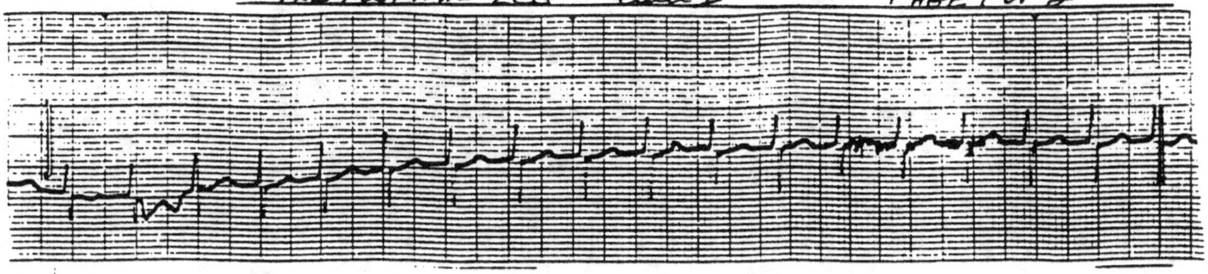

lead II

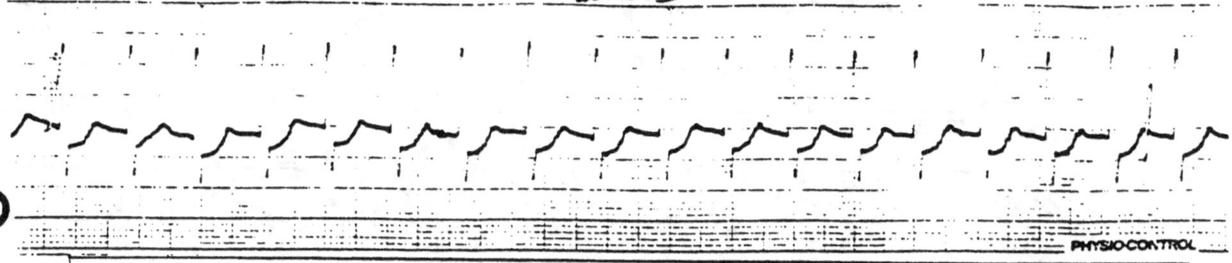

PHYSIO-CONTROL

lead III

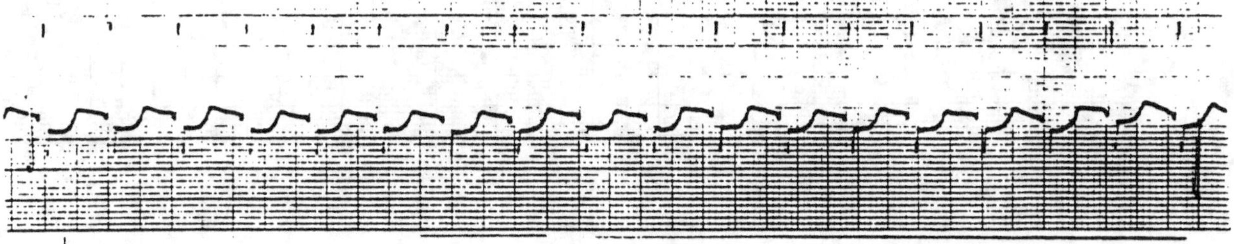

lead MCL I

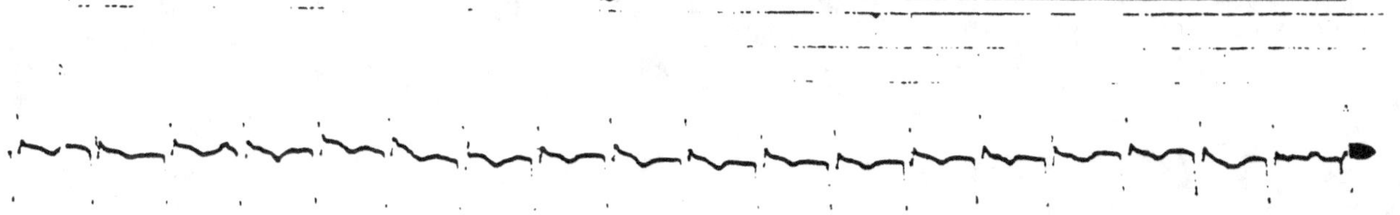

Trip #045 page 2 of 2

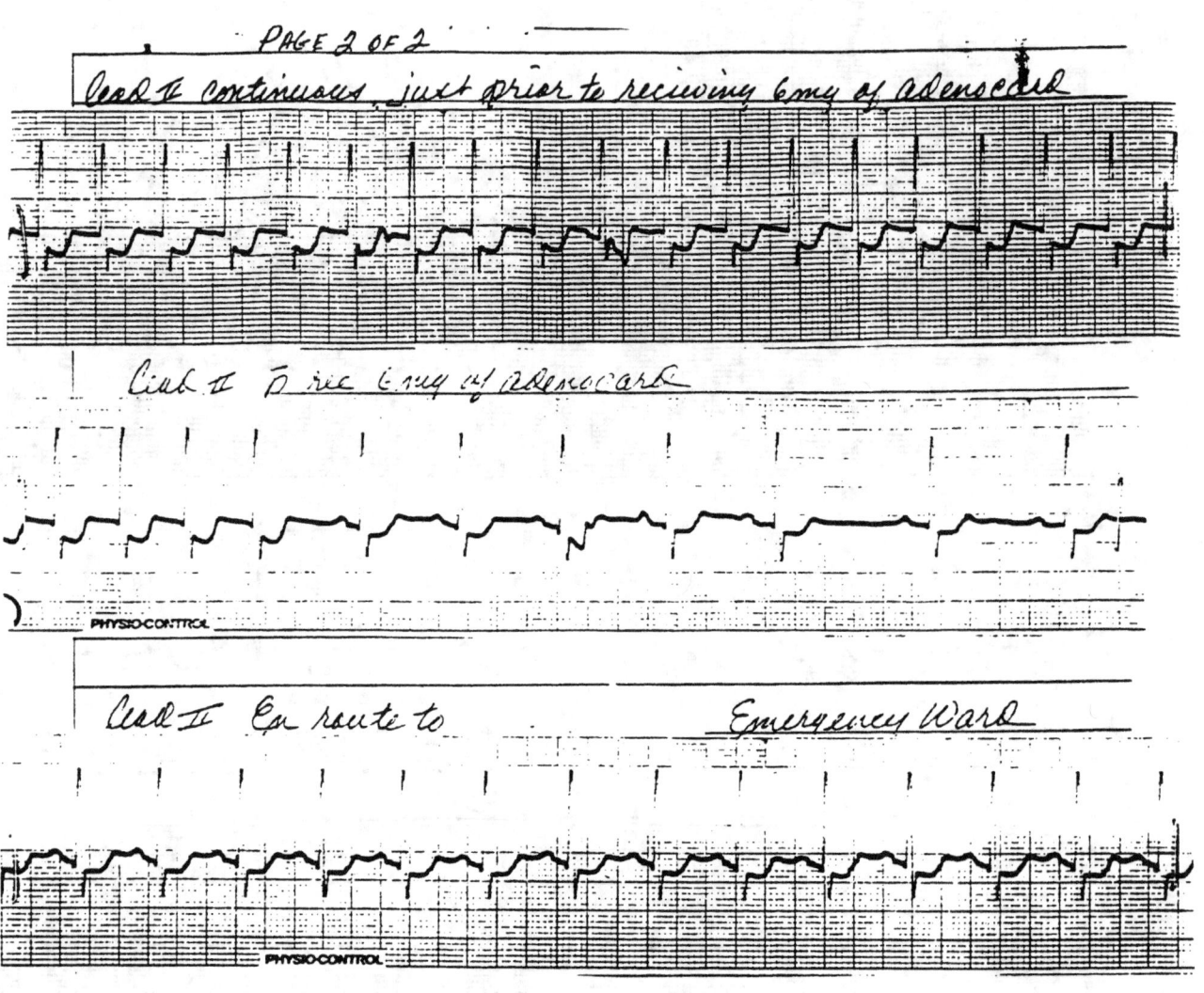

PAGE 2 OF 2

Lead II continuous, just prior to recieving 6mg of adenocard

Lead II To rec 6 mg of adenocard

PHYSIO-CONTROL

Lead II En route to   Emergency Ward

PHYSIO-CONTROL

12

Classroom Exercises

The following cases were developed from run reports completed by EMS personnel. Information that could potentially identify the patient has been changed.

This section is designed for participants to sort through information and organize it into a written report.

At the discretion of the instructor, students may work on the cases individually or in groups. Alternatively, classroom discussion can be developed around each case. When reviewing the reports that you write about each case, use questions such as:

1. What are the strengths reflected in this report?

2. What areas need improvement?

3. Does the report use the SEMS format being taught in this course?

4. Does the report clearly document the important points in the case?

5. Is the report a good medical record?

6. Is the report a good legal record?

7. Is is clear to you what occurred on the call?

8. Are times recorded?

9. Are all the necessary spaces filled in?

Cases

These cases are drawn from actual situations and reports, and can be used either for individual or group learning. The program is designed for use in either a BLS system, an ALS system, or a two-tiered system. The cases all have BLS parts. Some cases also continue with ALS intervention. Participants in this training program should write their report consistent with their level of training and certification.

Case 1, A cardiac patient

At the health unit of a local firm, a man walks in at the beginning of the day. He is complaining of a sense of heaviness in his chest. The medical unit personnel note that his skin coloration appears slightly pale. He is diaphoretic and a bit short of breath. The patient is visibly upset by the incident and has a look of concern, bordering on fear.

He tells them that he felt fine when he got up to go to work. The sensation of heaviness has only been present for about 20 minutes. He has never experienced anything like this before and he also feels as if he is going to throw up.

A quick check of his medical record reveals a history of hypertension that he is trying to control by diet. The man, a middle-management person about 48 years old, confirms that he does not take any prescription medications and does not have any known allergies.

A check of his vital signs by the nurse on duty yields a blood pressure of 190/120, and a pulse rate of 88. His skin coloration improves a bit, and he has stopped sweating. The decision is made to transport the gentleman to an emergency room, and an ambulance is called for. He is placed on oxygen by mask.

You respond at 7:35 A.M., and you arrive at 7:44 A.M. The building security staff directs you to the medical unit. You note the gentleman is in a supine position on a bed, jacket off and tie loosened. He manages a weak smile as you approach him, but the effort does little to mask the apprehension that he is feeling.

He recounts the story again saying he felt fine on the way to work. This sensation came on suddenly while he was at his desk. He also describes how his hands have this feeling of heaviness. Further questioning reveals that he has not eaten anything today, except a glass of juice before leaving the house. He still feels as if he could vomit but does not feel short of breath anymore.

The man says that his hypertension has not been controlled well by diet. He is considering medication to bring it under control. In fact, he has an appointment with his doctor later in the week.

You recheck the vital signs, noting that he has a BP of 184/116, a pulse rate of 75, and respiratory rate of 18/minute without dyspnea. The patient remains alert and oriented. His skin is warm and dry and there is no JVD. His breath sounds are equal and clear bilaterally. His abdomen is soft and non-tender, and he displays full use of all extremities. The sensation of heaviness in the chest is not altered by palpation or deep inspiration. You maintain him on a non-rebreather mask at 15 liters per minute.

BLS personnel may stop at this point except to record significant times and vital signs that are noted in the following paragraphs. Paramedics should continue with the case.

You obtain an ECG (see figure), and prepare the patient for transport. While doing this, your partner starts an I.V. of D_5W with an 18g angiocath to run at K.V.O. and draws bloods. You contact medical control and receive an order to give the patient a metered sub-lingual spray of nitroglycerine 0.4 mg. It is 8:04 A.M.

On a scale of 1 to 10, with 10 being the worse pain today, he describes the pain as a 10/10 before the nitroglycerine, and now a 5/10 after the nitroglycerine. His blood pressure is 164/70 and his pulse is 80 beats per minute, regular and full.

You move him down to the ambulance and at 8:06 A.M. you are enroute to the hospital. You repeat the nitroglycerine spray after 5 minutes. After the second administration of nitroglycerine 0.4 mg via sublingual spray, he describes the pain as a 3/10. He is not dyspneic. You arrive at the hospital before trying any further intervention. It is 8:12 A.M. His blood pressure during transport to the hospital is 176/P. His pulse is 75. His respiratory rate is 18. There is no dyspnea and his skin is warm and dry.

Case 2, A respiratory patient

Mrs. Smith has been worried about her husband's health for some time now. His difficulty with breathing, which he has had for several years, just gets worse.

Today, he awoke with trouble breathing and it is getting worse. He has lung problems. She knows that his heart is not doing that well either. He is sitting in a chair in the kitchen with all that he can do to catch his breath. Mrs. Smith realizes that she had better call an ambulance and get him to a hospital.

Your ambulance is dispatched at 0815 hours, and arrives eight minutes later. Mrs. Smith thinks that it took forever, but then she realizes that only a few minutes has passed since she called 911.

You begin to assess Mr. Smith, a 75 year old gentleman, noting that his color is pale. He is using a large amount of effort to breath. Mrs. Smith states that her husband has been sick like this before. She thinks that the cancer that was recently found in his right lung is making matters worse.

She hands your partner the list of medications that the hospital gave her to keep for her husband. He is taking Procardia®, isosorbide, Percocet®, theophylline, and Edecrin®.

Mr. Smith continues to concentrate all of his efforts on breathing. His lips are pursed and he is pale and diaphoretic. He is using his accessory muscles to help with breathing. When spoken to, he looks, but does not verbalize any response.

You get a set of vital signs. The blood pressure is 220/110. The pulse is 140/minute, and the respiratory rate is 40/minute. Mr. Smith displays severe dyspnea. A check of his lungs sounds reveals some sounds that are similar to rales, but are not clearly rales due to the wheezing that is occurring. The sounds are more prominent on the left side and extend from the bases towards the apices. His ankles also appear swollen.

You give Mr. Smith oxygen via non-rebreather at 12 liters per minute. Then you make a plan to extricate him from the house while treatment is continued.

As you are leaving, Mr. Smith's daughter arrives. She starts talking about how she really does not want any heroic efforts made on her father's behalf. She further states that he looked like this a few days ago. That was the last time he was brought to the hospital. She then gets into her automobile and as she drives away she announces that she will meet the ambulance at the hospital.

BLS personnel may stop at this point except to record significant times and vital signs that are noted in the next paragraph. Paramedics should continue with the case.

The total on-scene time has been 12 minutes. Two minutes before leaving for the hospital, you start an I.V. of D₅W, draw bloods and contact medical control. While enroute to the hospital you give nitroglycerine 0.4 mg by metered sublingual spray, and Lasix® 40 mg IVP. The patient's condition is getting worse, and you give morphine sulfate 2 mg IVP. Current blood pressure is 190/P, pulse is 140, and the respiratory rate is 40 per minute. There is increasing respiratory effort. The patient looks very tired. You prepare to intubate him. At 0841 hours you give nitroglycerine 0.8 mg via sublingual spray, repeat the morphine sulfate and intubate him. At 0845 hours you arrive at the hospital. The last vital sign check is BP 206/P, pulse 140, respirations assisted with bag valve mask via ET tube at 24 per minute.

Case 3, A trauma patient after a motor vehicle accident

It is 0800 hours. You are starting work on the day shift. You respond to a report of a motor vehicle overturned on a major highway. You arrive four minutes later, before any other responding agencies. A Jeep, equipped with a hardtop, is on its side in the breakdown lane. Several police officers arrive moments after you. They help you with the extrication.

Witnesses tell you that the vehicle was proceeding about 60 to 65 MPH when it was cut off by another vehicle. It rolled over multiple times through the lanes on the highway, and spun around. It is now resting on the driver's side facing oncoming traffic.

The driver, the sole occupant, is seated with his leg under the steering wheel. His right chest is wedged up against the side of the seat and the roof of the Jeep. His eyes are open and he is looking around. The entire extrication process takes 10 minutes, and you are enroute to the hospital 4 minutes after that, arriving there eight minutes later.

He is about 35 years old, conscious, very anxious looking, and unable to speak. After calming him down a bit, he can tell you his name and that he remembers being in an accident. He has good skin coloration with slightly moist skin. His pupils are equal at 5 mm and reactive to light. He complains of pain to his neck on the left side, and his left clavicle and shoulder. His trachea is midline. There is no obvious deformity to his neck and chest and the chest wall moves symmetrically. His breath sounds are equal but he cannot take a deep breath because it hurts. His abdomen is soft, he complains of pain to the left groin with femoral pulses present and symmetrical. He displays good motor and sensory function as well as distal pulses in the extremities. He has good bilateral grip.

Vital signs are: BP 180/100; Pulse 100; RR 22 shallow.

The extrication is accomplished with the patient being immobilized on a backboard with precautions taken for cervical, thoracic and lumbar spinal injuries. His legs are also splinted.

He is maintained on oxygen via non-rebreather at 15 liters per minute.

For paramedics: As you are leaving the scene, an I.V. of normal saline solution is started at a KVO rate using a 14g angiocath in the right fossa.

Case 4, A gun shot wound

It is a mid-autumn evening. At 2300 hours you respond to a parking lot for a report of a person shot. Your arrival coincides with that of the police, at 2304 hours. A small crowd has gathered around a 25 year-old male who is on the ground. The lot is poorly lit. You note that he still is breathing. His eyes open when people speak to him. He is moving his legs.

As you get closer you hear the story that a couple of shots were fired from a moving vehicle into a group that was gathered in the lot. The patient tells you that he has been shot. He is very anxious.

A quick exam reveals evidence of bleeding from the chest area. You move the patient into the ambulance and conduct a more thorough examination. Four minutes after arriving at the call, you are enroute to the hospital.

There is no evidence of head trauma. Pupils are dilated but react to light. You note a slight odor of alcohol. The neck veins are flat, the chest wall moves symmetrically. There is a wound at the left costal arch on the anterior axillary line. The breath sounds are present bilaterally. They are clear on the right side, with some diminished sound on the left side.

Continuing the exam, you find another wound in the abdomen in the left lower quadrant. The femoral pulses are present and symmetrical. There is no evidence of trauma to the lower extremities. When you roll the patient, an exit wound is visible in the left posterior abdomen. The patient is moving his arms and legs on his own.

Vital signs are: BP 86/50; Pulse 140, weak, regular; RR 28 shallow. The patient looks up at you and asks you if he is going to die.

The ride to the hospital takes ten minutes. *For paramedics:* You start an I.V. of normal saline to run wide open through a 16g angiocath in the left fossa. You do this just after leaving the scene. A repeat set of vital signs is obtained. The blood pressure is 98/P, pulse 120, regular, 1⁺ at the radial, and respirations are regular though still shallow at 28 per minute.

Case 5, A pediatric patient

It is 9:30 A.M. You respond to the rear of a home were a child has fallen. You arrive 5 minutes later. In the back yard you see a 9 year old boy who has fallen from a 1' wall and has an obvious deformity to the left lower leg.

His mother tells you that he was playing outside and she heard him yell for her.

As you speak with the boy, you note that he responds well to your questions. He is in obvious pain. He cries occasionally as you examine him. You find there is no injury to his head. He tells you that he did not hit his head. There is lack of pain or tenderness to his neck. His chest and abdomen do not have any signs of injury, and his breath sounds are equal and clear. He has a soft abdomen. It is not tender to the touch. He does not have any back pain.

There are some minor abrasions to his arms and legs. The left leg has an angulation at the lower ⅓ of the tibia. He can feel you touch his feet, but he will not move his left foot or toes because it hurts too much. The muscles of his left lower leg are very tense. Both feet are warm to the touch, and the pulses in the feet are symmetrical.

As you stabilize the leg, your partner brings splinting material. The two of you splint the leg and place him on the stretcher. You elevate the leg slightly, and transport him to the hospital.

Your on-scene time is 8 minutes.

While on the way to the hospital his mother tells you that he is a healthy child without any significant medical problems. He does not take any medications regularly. He does get hay fever in the Fall.

You arrive at the hospital after a 10 minute ride. There is no change in the condition of the patient.

Case 6, A diabetic (hypoglycemia)

You receive a call to respond to an office building for an unconscious person. You arrive at the building, are escorted to the elevator, and are brought to the 5th floor reception area. A group of people are gathered around a 36 year old woman who is laid out across a couch.

The co-workers tell you that the woman was not acting in her usual manner, she became weak and dizzy, and she was helped by them to the couch. They further tell you that the woman has a history of diabetes. She does not usually have any problems with it. They have given her some orange juice, but it took a lot of coaxing to get her to drink anything. They did get her to take a glucose tablet. As you begin your exam of the patient, another co-worker states that the patient has just returned from having a mammogram done.

You findings are that the patient has a sluggish response to her name, but does open her eyes and look at you. She is non-diaphoretic. You do not see any evidence of trauma. There is no JVD, the breath sounds are equal and clear, and the abdomen is soft. Your partner gets the following vital signs: BP 130/80 Pulse 80 and regular, and respirations are 20 per minute with normal depth and effort.

Her husband has been contacted by telephone. He reports that his wife is an insulin dependent diabetic. She does not take any other medications and does not have any known allergies. He further states that he is on the way from his office, located about 10 to 15 minutes away.

Your partner tells you that the patient's mental status is improving. The husband wants to take the patient home instead of to a hospital. As you speak with him, you note that the patient is becoming oriented to her surroundings. She is saying that she does not want to go to a hospital.

Case 7, A cardiac arrest

It is 10:00 in the morning. While driving on a downtown street, a citizen flags you down and brings you to a person who has just collapsed inside a municipal building. It takes you two minutes to get to the patient.

CPR is in progress. The man is about 70 years old, and is exhibiting agonal respirations. He does not have a pulse. The ECG shows him to be in ventricular fibrillation. You provide a countershock at 200 joules. He is still in pulseless V-F, so you countershock him again, this time at 300 joules. He first goes to pulseless asystole, then to a pulseless rhythm at 20 to 30 complexes per minute. He rapidly develops a perfusing rhythm with a pulse of 40, BP 84/66, and an occasional respiratory effort. It is now 4 minutes since you were first flagged down at the building.

You have now been with the patient a total of five minutes. As you try to start an I.V. and to intubate the patient, he develops pulseless V-F. You countershock at 300 joules, he again develops a perfusing rhythm. This time his blood pressure is 80/P, pulse 120, with some occasional respiratory effort. You start an I.V. at a point 10 minutes after your first arrival with the patient. You give lidocaine 100 mg IVP, start a Lidocaine infusion, and contact medical control for orders on the drip rate for the I.V. At this point you are moving the patient out to the ambulance. The order is for Lidocaine 2 mg/minute.

You start a second I.V. and run in a 200 cc Bolus of normal saline. The patient is making increased respiratory effort. He resists attempts to orally intubate, so you nasotracheally intubate the patient with a 6.0 mm E.T. tube and assist his respirations. As you leave for the hospital his BP is 168/120, pulse is 100. You are running the saline line at KVO.

During the 3 minute ride to the hospital, you check his blood pressure. It is 160/P. His pulse is 110, and he is still making some effort to breath. You continue assisting with ventilations. Total time of the call from when you were flagged down to arrival at the hospital is 34 minutes.

Case 8, A seizure patient

It is 1100 hours. You are in a BLS ambulance. You respond to a report of an elderly person "not looking too good." You arrive at 1108 hours. A family member meets you at the door to a multi-unit apartment building and you walk up to the third floor. There you find an elderly woman slumped over in a chair.

The initial exam shows her to be breathing rapidly with some noise. She has a fast pulse. She is not responding to either you or the family members.

As your partner takes a set of vital signs and does a physical exam, you interview the family. They tell you that the patient has been in good health. There is some discussion amongst them about diabetes. You are told that whatever that was, it was years ago. The patient does not take any medications and the family members are not aware of any allergies that the patient has. You are also told that it has been a while since the patient has been seen by a doctor.

You partner informs you that the vital signs are: BP 184/84, Pulse is 160, and the respiratory rate is 36 and shallow. The skin is hot to the touch. The patient has breath sounds present bilaterally, with the right side clearer that the left. The left also sounds a bit distant. The abdomen is soft to the touch, without any evidence of distension. There is no evidence of any trauma. You give the patient oxygen via non-rebreather mask at 15 liters per minute.

As you begin to move the patient, she starts seizing. At this point you note that the pupils are equal and are about 2 mm in diameter. The eyes deviate to the right.

BLS personnel may stop at this point except to record significant times and vital signs that are noted in the next paragraph, as well as what their treatment would be after the changes in patient condition occur. Paramedics should continue with the case.

Your paramedic unit arrives on scene. The EMTs give you a report on the patient. At 11:55 A.M. you start an I.V. of normal saline to run at KVO, and draw bloods. Your partner does a dextrose level check, and the chemstrip reads 200 mg/dl. Within 3 minutes of this you give thiamine 100 mg IVP and naloxone 1 mg IVP. The seizures remain uncontrolled.

Within ten minutes after the initial I.V. start, you give the patient Valium 5 mg IVP, and then orally intubate her with a 7.0 mm endotracheal tube. The patient is in respiratory arrest. You assist the respirations. She is still seizing. You repeat the Valium 5 mg IVP 10 minutes after the first administration. As you do this you are enroute to the hospital.

While enroute, the patient stops seizing, her blood pressure takes a sudden drop to 90/60, and the pulse rate is 110. The patient is still in respiratory arrest. You open the normal saline wide, giving a 250 cc bolus. Within 2 minutes of the bolus administration the patient's BP is 102/70. You arrive at the hospital without any further change in the patient.

Special Situations

Case 9, Is it a medical or a police matter?

It is 3:30 in the afternoon. Your BLS unit responds to a restaurant in a hotel. A member of the hotel security directs you into the lounge area beside the restaurant. You see an adult male wearing a sport coat and tie. He is about in his mid-forties. The gentleman is seated at the bar. He does not acknowledge your presence. Hotel security informs you that the bartender summoned them. He was concerned by the behavior of the man. According to the bartender, he does not look well.

The bartender tells you the following story: The man has been seated for about two hours. In that time, he has ordered two drinks. He consumed the first. The second is visible in front of him, virtually untouched. He has not been conversing, even when conversation is directed his way. Mostly, he stares ahead, expressionless. Occasionally, he adjusts his position but he has not moved from the seat.

The bartender is concerned by the behavior. It is inconsistent with the surroundings, not characteristic with what he normally sees. He therefore felt that help should be summoned. He further relates that the man did not appear intoxicated when he first arrived in the lounge.

The local police department has also arrived on the scene and you quickly tell them the story.

You approach the man and ask him what is wrong. He proceeds to clench the edge of the bar with his fists and to breathe in a noisy and rapid manner. He then calms down. You ask him again. He does not reply, just turns his head to look at you. You ask his name. Without warning he jumps from the seat, assumes a martial arts position, and threatens you.

In the following scuffle, he is restrained without apparent injury.

Background information for the case:

The man is not incontinent. He is non-diaphoretic, does not converse, and is not wearing a medic alert tag. There is no evidence of prior injury, drug abuse, intoxication or seizure activity. Neither blood pressure nor pulse can be accurately obtained due to the thrashing about of the patient. From all outward appearances, he is a businessman having a late afternoon cocktail.

Questions—Case 9

Will the patient be treated as a medical emergency or a police matter?

1. If you decide it is a police matter, do you need to write a report?

   If you think you need a report, write the report. If you think you do not need to write a report, write a rationale for this decision on a separate piece of paper.

2. If you decide it is a medical emergency, do you need to write a report?

   If you think you need a report, write the report. If you think you do not need to write a report, write a rationale for this decision on a separate piece of paper.

3. If you are a paramedic, and responded to this call in an ALS unit, would you handle the situation differently? Explain your answer.

Case 10, How would you write it?

It is 10:30 at night. You respond to a motor vehicle accident. The scene is that of a single automobile into a tree. There is only one occupant. The patient appears intoxicated, as indicated by the odor of alcohol.

You try to immobilize this conscious patient on a backboard. You start the procedure, then the patient refuses treatment. You decide to remove the backboard and cervical collar.

Discussion: The odor of alcohol suggests impaired mental status and the inability to foresee the results of one's actions. The problem becomes one of either fighting with the patient, who has a potential back injury, thus aggravating the injury, or removing the splinting material with the resultant destabilization of the potential back injury.

What should be documented and how should it be written? Write the report showing that you removed the board and collar under the circumstances stated in the case.

Case 11, What would you do?

It is 2:00 PM. You are in a BLS unit responding to a report of a person who has collapsed at home. Family members tell you that the patient collapsed and was on the floor gasping. They immediately called the ambulance. Your total response time was about six minutes. Total time from the patient's collapse to the arrival of your ambulance is 9 to 11 minutes.

The patient presents lying on the floor by the front door. The relative says that the patient, a male about 70 years old, is without a pulse. Your initial examination shows a patient with no respiration, no pulse and dilated pupils. His hands are half-clenched and cold. You are told by the family that the patient had been to the doctor the night before. He has a history of heart problems and maybe a stroke.

• What will you do from this point?

• Will you resuscitate or not?

Write your report based on whether you would resuscitate or not, then be prepared to present the rationale for your decision. If you choose to resuscitate, write a BLS report documenting transport to the hospital with the care you would give. If you choose not to resuscitate, write a BLS report documenting the decision.

Case 12, A sudden death

It is 7:00 A.M. You respond to a call to help with an unresponsive person in a single family home. The family meets you at the door when you arrive 7 minutes later. They are somewhat panicky and distraught as they bring you to the bedroom where an elderly female is lying on the bed. As you quickly check the patient, you note that she is cool to the touch and pale to cyanotic in color. Her eyes are open and are not blinking. She is not breathing and does not have a pulse. There is some stiffness to her neck.

One of the family members says to you "She's gone, isn't she?"

You ask what happened this morning, and they tell you that their grandmother is usually up around 5:30 A.M. to 6:00 A.M. Today she did not get up. After a time, when they did not hear any movement in her bedroom, they went in to check on her. They found her as you see her now.

They provide you with a box full of medications when you ask about her medical history. The box contains Bumex®, digoxin nitroglycerine 1 / 150 gr, hydrochlorothiazide, and propranolol.

She was not allergic to anything that they know of.

Her physician is Dr. Reed.

The police officer who was sent on the call with you has arrived while you were interviewing the family. You explain the situation to her. You write a report and call the medical examiner, according to your system protocol. You leave a copy of the report with the police officer, extend your condolences to the family, and leave.

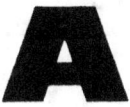

Common Deficiencies
in Report Writing

Leaving blank spaces

Examples:

- Not filling in times.
- Not recording the time when vital signs were taken.
- Not noting delivery device and rate/route when giving oxygen.
- Not showing treatment given.
- Not recording the mileage.
- Not recording the assessment findings. Not noting the treatment given.

Other points

- Record the dispatch address.
- Record the nature code.
- Get the name and address of the patient.
- Describe the situation, give a good picture of the history.
- Use standard abbreviations.
- Any jargon must be consistent within the occupation.

- If using abbreviations, they have to be common knowledge abbreviations, not something made up by the EMT or paramedic.

- Organize thoughts before writing.

- Remember that billing information is also important, even in the public sector.

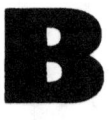

105 CMR 170.240
Records

Every ambulance service shall be responsible for the preparation and maintenance of records which are subject to and shall be available for inspection by the Department upon request. Records shall be stored in such a manner as to insure reasonable safety from water and fire damage and from unauthorized use for a period of not less than three (3) years.

(B) Trip records shall be maintained for all ambulance runs and shall at a minimum include date, times, location of dispatch, pickup and delivery, relevant patient information, including medical condition at scene and in transit, names of attendants, and identification of vehicle.

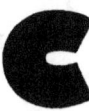

Mass. Department of Public Health/ Office of Emergency Medical Services Process for Investigating ——————— Complaints

Anyone can file a complaint through any means. Complaints can be anonymous. The law requires the Department to investigate all complaints. The first step is to pull the run report. The first question then asked is if there is a need to investigate. If the documentation is good, the investigation could start and end right there. It is entirely possible that under a circumstance such as this the EMTs or paramedics involved may not know of the investigation.

However, most cases do not have good documentation, so the investigation goes to the next step. This involves interviewing the parties involved and getting written statements about the incident. After the parties involved read the statements, they can make changes and corrections. Then they sign and date the statements. A peer review of the case follows. At this point there are three options. Either it becomes a closed case, has a hearing scheduled, or has more information gathered.

The Department of Public Health issues reprimands at this point. Reprimands at this point mean you gave poor care. Despite the poor care, you did not harm the patient.. If minor harm was done, there may be grounds for suspension. If major harm was done, they see you as a public health threat. Your certificate is subject to revocation.

Public Health sends notices concerning hearings. The respondent has seven days in which to reply. They appoint a hearing officer to conduct the hearing. After the hearing, the public health council votes on an action. Usually, they agree with the hearing officer. Any appeal of the action is through the court system.

Abandonment: Abrupt ending of contact with the patient. The patient is not given enough opportunity to find another health professional to take over his medical treatment, or is left in the hands of less-trained providers.[82]

Breach of Duty: Action measured against that of an average performing reputable member of the provider's peer group. Identify average medical knowledge and professional performance in the peer group. When measured against the average, the action it is inconsistent with the accepted standard of conduct. Negligence occurred.[83]

Consent, Actual: Consent actually given by a person. May be oral or in writing.[84]

Consent, Implied: Consent shown by an individual voluntarily entered a situation.[85] In some emergency situations, actual consent is unobtainable. The law assumes the patient consents to limited life-saving actions.[86]

Consent, Informed: Consent given by a person who understands the nature and extent of the proposed procedure. The person then agrees to having the procedure done. The person has enough mental and physical capacity to make such a judgment.[87]

Consent: Agreement by the patient to accept a medical intervention.[88]

Duty to Act: Legal obligation of public and other ambulance services. They must respond to calls for help in their jurisdiction.[89]

Duty to Perform: Exists when the patient presents to the health care organization and its members as in need of emergency care. The provider has a duty to perform in the best interest of the patient. This duty establishes itself when the patient first presents as in need of care.[90]

Malpractice: Incorrect or negligent treatment of a patient occurs by persons responsible for health care.[91]

Negligence: The healthcare provider fails to perform an important or necessary technique. Also, performing such a technique in a careless or unskilled manner that results in further injury.[92]

Standard of Care: The usual or accepted manner of giving care in effect at the time. This includes the actions and behavior of the health care provider.[93]

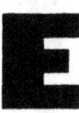

Commonly-Used Abbreviations

A text on documentation should contain a list of standard abbreviations. This text is no different. Including the list is, however, not without some risk.

Any list of abbreviations will be incomplete. There are always obscure abbreviations. Also, an abbreviation may be well-accepted in one region, and virtually unheard of in another. Furthermore, including the list may tempt the user to turn his written reports into an alphabet soup of run-on abbreviations, the result being utter confusion on the part of the reader.

The list is useful as a guide. It was developed from several sources. It contains abbreviations likely to be used or encountered by EMS personnel. If you encounter abbreviations not listed here, remember that the reference texts contain more complete lists. Also, referring to a medical dictionary might be helpful.

ø	None	AAL	Anterior axillary line
a, ā	Ante (before)	ab	Abortion
A	Anorexia, aorta, artery, auscultation, albumin	abd	Abdominal
		ABD	Abdomen, abduction
a.d.	Right ear	ABE	Acute bacterial endocarditis
A.P.	Apical pulse	ABG	Arterial blood gas
a.s.	Left ear	ABGs	Arterial blood gases
a.u.	Both ears	ac	Ante cibum (before meals)
AAA	Abdominal aortic aneurysm	ACh	Acetylcholine

ACLS	Advanced cardiac life support		bilat	Bilateral
ad	To or toward		BKA	Below-the-knee amputation
ADH	Antidiuretic hormone		BLS	Basic life support
AF	Atrial fibrillation, aorto-femoral		BM	Bowel movement, black man, black male
AI	Aortic insufficiency		BO	Body odor
AKA	Above-the-knee amputation		BP	Blood pressure
α	Alpha		BRB	Bright red blood
ALS	Advanced life support		BS	Bowel sounds, breath sounds, blood smear, blood sugar
AMA	Against medical advice		BUN	Blood urea nitrogen
amb	Ambulance		BW	Black woman
AMI	Acute (or anterior) myo-cardial infarction		C	Celsius
amp	Ampule		C&F	Chills and fever
AP	Anteroposterior, angina pectoris, acid phosphatase		c, c̄	With
ARDS	Adult respiratory distress syndrome		C-Spine	Cervical spine
ARF	Acute rheumatic fever, acute renal failure		C/C/E	Clubbing/cyanosis/edema
AS	Aortic stenosis, arterio-sclerosis		c/o	Complains of
ASA	Aspirin		CA	Cancer, cardiac arrest
ASAP	As soon as possible		Ca	Calcium
AV	Arteriovenous, atrioven-tricular		Ca++	Calcium ion
AVB	Atrioventricular block		CABG	Coronary artery bypass graft(ing)
AVN	Atrioventricular node		$CaCl_2$	Calcium chloride
AVR	Aortic valve replacement		CAD	Coronary artery disease
ax	Axillary		CAH	Chronic active hepatitis
B&J, B + J	Bone and joint		cap	Capsule
BB	Bundle branch		caps	Capsules
BBB	Bundle-branch block		CAT	Computerized axial tomography (an x-ray)
β	Beta		CBC	Complete blood count
BF	Black female		cc, CC	Chief complaint, cubic centimeter
BFB	Bifascicular block		CCJ	Costochondral junction
bid, b.i.d.	Bis in diem (twice a day)		CDB	Cough and deep-breathe
			CF	Caucasian female, cystic fibrosis
			CHD	Congenital heart disease

CHF	Congestive heart failure	$D_{50}W$	50% dextrose in water
Cl	Chloride	D_5W	5% dextrose in water
Cl–	Chloride ion	DC	Discontinue; discharge
CM	Caucasian man, Caucasian male	Ddx	Differential diagnosis
cm	Centimeter	DI	Diabetes insipidus
cm^3	Cubic centimeter	diff	Difficulty
CNS	Central nervous system	dig., Dig	digitalis
CO	Carbon monoxide	DJD	Degenerative joint disease
CO_2	Carbon dioxide	DKA	Diabetic ketoacidosis
COLD	Chronic obstructive lung disease	DM	Diabetes mellitus
Cor	Heart	DOA	Dead on arrival
CP	Chest pain, cerebral palsy	DOB	Date of birth
CPAP	Continuous positive airway pressure	DOE	Dyspnea on exertion
CPR	Cardiopulmonary resuscitation	DP	Dorsalis pedis (pulse)
CR	Cardiorespiratory	DPH	Diphenylhydantoin (phenytoin) (Dilantin)
Cr	Creatinine	DPT	Diphtheria, pertussis, tetanus (immunization)
CRD	Chronic respiratory disease	DS	Disease
CRF	Chronic renal failure	dsg	Dressing
CSF	Cerebrospinal fluid	DTRs	Deep tendon reflexes
CSM	Carotid sinus massage	DTs	Delerium tremens
CT	Computerized tomography	DU	Duodenal ulcer
CV	Cardiovascular	Dx	Diagnosis
CVA	Costovertebral angle, cerebrovascular accident	E&R	Equal and reactive
CVP	Central venous pressure	EBL	Estimated blood loss
CW	Caucasian woman	ECG	Electrocardiogram
/d	Day, daily	ECT	Electroconvulsive therapy
dl	Deciliter	EEG	Electroencephalogram
D&C	Dilation and curettage	EKG	Electrocardiogram
D&W	Dextrose in water	elix	Elixir
D.M.	Diabetes mellitus	EMT	Emergency medical treatment (or triage, or technician)
D.O.	Doctor of osteopathic medicine	ENT	Ear, nose, and throat
D/C	Discontinued, discharged	EOA	Esophageal obturator airway
D/NS	Dextrose and normal saline	EOAG	EOA with gastric tube

EOM	Extraocular motions (EOMI = EOM intact; EOMF = EOM full)
ER	Emergency room
ERV	Expiratory reserve volume
est	Estimated
ET	Endotracheal
et.	And
ETA	Estimated time of arrival
ETOH	Ethyl alcohol
ETT	Endotracheal tube
EW	Emergency ward
F	Fever, female, Fahrenheit
F°	Degrees Fahrenheit
FB, F.B.	Foreign body
FBS	Fasting blood surgar
Fe	Iron
FEV	Forced expiratory volume
FG	Fasting glucose
FH	Family history
FLB	(funny looking beats) Usually premature ventricular ventricular beats. May be supraventricular beats with aberrant QRS conduction.
Flds	Fluids
FROM	Full range of motion
FTT	Failure to thrive
FUO	Fever of unknown origin
Fx, FX	Fracture
g, G	Gram
G.T.T.	Glucose tolerance test
GB	Gallbaldder
GBD	Gallbaldder disease
GC	Gonorrhea (from gonococcus)
GE	Gastroenteritis
Gen	Generally, genitalia
GI	Gastrointestinal

Gl	Gland, glucose
gm	Gram
GP	General practitioner, general paresis (tertiary neurosyphilis)
gr	Grain
GSW	Gunshot wound
gtt(s), Gtt	Guttae (drops)
GU	Genitourinary
gyn, GYN	Gynecology, gynecologic
h	Hour
H&P	History and physical
h/a, HA	Headache
HBP	High blood pressure
Hct	Hematocrit
HCTZ	Hydrochlorothiazide
HEENT	Head, ears, eyes, nose, throat
Heme	Blood, hematology
Hg	Mercury
Hgb	Hemoglobin
HO	House officer
Hosp	Hospital
HPI	History of present illness
HR	Heart rate
Ht	Height
HTN	Hypertension
Hx	History
ICP	Intracranial pressure
ICS	Intercostal space
ID	Infectious disease
IDDM	Dependent
IH	Infectious hepatitis
IM	Intramuscular
Inf MI	Inferior myocardial infarction
IPPB	Intermittent positive pressure breathing

IRDM	Insulin-requiring diabetes mellitus		LLL	Left lower lobe, late latent lues
IU	International unit		LLQ	Lower left quadrant
IUD	Intrauterine device		LMP	Last menstrual period
IV	Intravenous		LOA	Level of activity, leave of absence
IVC	Intravenous cholangiogram, inferior vena cava		LOC	Loss of consciousness
IVP	IV push		LPHB	Left posterior hemiblock
IVPB	IV (intravenous) piggyback		LPN	Licensed practical nurse
JAR	Junior assistant resident		LR	Lactated Ringer's
JOD	Juvenile onset diabetes		LS	Lumbar spine
jt	Joint		LSB	Left sternal border
JVD	Jugular venous distention		LUE	Left upper extremity
JVP	Jugular venous pressure		LUL	Left upper lobe
K	Potassium, ketones		LUQ	Left upper quadrant
K^+	Potassium ion		LV	Left ventricle
kg	Kilogram		LVH	Left ventricular hypertrophy
(T)KO	(To) Keep open		LVN	Licensed vocational nurse
KVO	Keep vein open		m, Ⓜ	Murmur
L	Left, lymphocyte, lung, lobe		M.D.	Doctor of medicine
l, L	Liter		MAL	Midaxillary line
L&A	Light and accommodation		MBL	Minimal blood loss
L-Spine	Lumbar spine		MCL	Midclavicular line
LA	Left atrium, left arm, left anterior		med(s)	Medication(s)
lac	Laceration		mEq	Milliequivalent
LAD	Left axis deviation, left anterior descending (coronary artery)		Mg	Magnesium
			μg	Microgram
			mg	Milligram
LAH	Left anterior hemiblock		μm	Micrometer
LAHB	Left anterior hemiblock		MI	Mitral insufficiency, myocardial infarction
lb	Pound			
LBBB	Left bundle branch block		MICU	Medical intensive care unit
LBP	Low back pain		min	Minute
lg	Large		ML	Midline
LHF	Left heart failure		ml	Milliliter
Li	Lithium		mm	Millimeter
LLE	Left lower extremity		MOD	Maturity onset diabetes
			mod	Moderate

MS	Mitral stenosis; multiple sclerosis; morphine sulfate
MSL	Midsternal line
MSO_4	Morphine sulfate
mutl	Multiple
MVA	Motor vehicle accident
N&V	Nausea and vomiting
N_2O	Nitrous oxide
NA, N/A	No answer, not applicable
Na	Sodium
Na+	Sodium ion
NAD	No acute distress, no active disease
$NaHCO_3$	Sodium bicarbonate
nb	Newborn
NC, N/C	Nasal cannula; no charge
neg	Negative
NES	Not elsewhere specified
NF	Negro female
NG, N/G	Nasogastric
NIAL	Not in active labor
nitro	Nitroglycerin
NK	Not known, nonketonic
NKA	No known allergies
NKDA	No known drug allergies
Nl	Normal
NM	Negro man, Negro male
NMT	Nebulized mist treatments
NN	Nerves
noc	Night
NPO	Nothing by mouth
NR	Nonreactive, not relevant
NROM	Normal range of motion
NS	Normal saline
NS	Not sufficient
NSR	Normal sinus rhythm
NSVD	Normal spontaneous vaginal delivery

NT	Nasotracheal
NTG	Nitroglycerin
NVD	Nausea, vomiting, diarrhea
NW	Negro woman
O	Oxygen
o.d.	Right eye
o.s.	Left eye
o.u.	Each eye
O_2	Oxygen
OB	Obstetric(s)
OBS	Organic brain syndrome
occ	Occasional
OD	Overdose
OM	Otitis media
ONC	Oncology
OPD	Outpatient department
OPP	Organophosphate poisoning
OR	Operating room
Ortho	Orthopedics, orthostatic
OS	Opening snap, mouth, left eye (oculus sinister)
OT	Occupational therapy, oxaloacetic transaminase (SGOT)
oz	Ounce
p, $\bar{p}$	After, post
P&A	Percussion and auscultation
p.c.	After meals
P.E.	Pulmonary embolism, physical examination
P.O.	Postoperative
PA	Posteroanterior, physician's assistant, pulmonary artery, pernicious anemia
PAB	Premature atrial beat
PAC	Premature atrial contraction
PAF	Paroxysmal atrial fibrillation (or flutter)

PAP	Pulmonary artery pressure, Papanicolaou (cervical) smear
PAT	Paroxysmal atrial tachycardia
PB	Piggyback
PCN	Penicillin
PD	Police department
PE	Pulmonary edema, pulmonary embolus
ped	Pedestrian
pedi	Pediatric
PEEP	Positive end-expiratory pressure
PEN	Penicillin
PERL(A)	Pupils equal and reactive to light (and accommodation)
PERRLA	Pupils equal, round, react to light and accommodation
PH	Past history, pulmonary hypertension
PHx	Past history
PID	Pelvic inflammatory disease
PJC	Premature junctional contraction
PM	Post mortem
PMD, (LMD)	Private medical doctor
PMI	Point of maxium impulse
PND	Paroxysmal noctural dyspnea
PNH	Paroxysmal nocturnal hemoglobinuria
po, PO	Per os (by mouth)
poss	Possible
Post	Autopsy (used as noun)
PP	Postpartum
PPD	Purified proten derivative (tuberculosis skin test), percussion and postural drainage, pack per day (smoking)

pr, PR	Per rectum
prn	As necessary (pro re nata)
prox	Proximal
PSVT	Paroxysmal supraventricular tachycardia
PT	Physical therapy
pt	Patient
PTA	Prior to arrival (admission)
PVB	Premature ventricular beat
PVC	Premature ventricular contraction
$q, \overline{q}$	Quaque (each, every)
Q	Perfusion (blood flow)
qd	Every day
qh	Every hour
qid, q.i.d.	Four times a day
qod	Every other day
qs	Sufficient quantity
qt	Quart
Quad	Quadriplegic
R on T	A premature QRS beat falling on top of T wave from previous beat
R/O	Rule out
RA	Rheumatoid arthritis, right atrium, right arm, right anterior
RAD	Right axis deviation
RBBB	Right bundle-branch block
RBC(s)	Red blood cell(s)
RC	Roman Catholic, respirations ceased (died)
RDS	Respiratory disease syndrome; Respiratory distress syndrome
RE	Regional enteritis, right eye
req	Request
RF	Rheumatic fever, renal failure, respiratory failure, releasing factor

RICU	Respiratory intensive care unit
RL	Ringer's lactate
RLE	Right lower extremity
RLL	Right lower lobe
RLQ	Right lower quadrant
RML	Right middle lobe
ROJM	Range of joint motion
ROM	Range of motion
ROS	Review of symptoms
RPT	Registered physical therapist; repeat
RR	Respiratory rate
RSB	Right sternal border
RT	Respiration therapy
Rt	Routine
RUE	Right upper extremity
RUL	Right upper lobe
RUQ	Right upper quadrant
RV	Right ventricle; residual volume
RVH	Right ventricular hypertrophy
Rx	Treatment, therapy
s, $\bar{s}$	Without
S-Spine	Sacral spine
S/P	Status post (after)
S_1	First heart sound
S_2	Second heart sound
S_3	Third heart sound
S_4	Fourth heart sound
SA	Sinoatrial, septic arthritis
SAH	Subarachnoid hemorrhage
SAN	Sinoatrial node
SAR	Senior assistant resident
SB	Sinus bradycardia
SBO	Small bowel obstruction
SC	Subcutaneous(ly)
SCM	Sternocleidomastoid
SICU	Surgical intensive care unit
Sig:	Let it be labeled
SL	Sublingual
sl	Slight
sm	Small
SOB	Shortness of breath
sol., Sol	Solution
SQ	Subcutaneous(ly)
ss	Half
SSS	Sick sinus syndrome
stat, STAT	Now or immediately
sub q, SubQ	Subcutaneous(ly)
Supp	Suppository
SVC	Superior vena cava
SVT	Supraventricular tachycardia
SW	Stab wound
Sx/Sx	Signs and symptoms
Syr	Syrup
T	Temperature, time
T&C	Type and cross (blood)
T-Spine	Thoracic
TA, TAb	Therapeutic abortion
Tab	Tablet
TB	Tuberculosis
TFB	Trifascicular block
TIA	Transient ischemic attack
TICU	Thoracic intensive care unit
tid, t.i.d.	Three times a day
TKO	To keep open
TLC	Total lung capacity; tender loving care
TMJ	Temporomandibular joint
TPR	Temperature, pulse, respiration
tr	Tincture
TT	Transtracheal

Tx	Transport		VNA	Visiting Nurse Association
u.	Unit		VO	Verbal orders
u.d.	As directed		VS	Vital signs
UE	Upper extremities		VSS	Vital signs stable
UH	University hospital		VT	Ventricular tachycardia
Unc	Unconscious		VW	Veins
UQ	Upper quadrant		W/C	Wheelchair
URI	Upper respiratory tract infection		W/D	Withdrawal
ut. dict.	As directed		W/O	Without
UTI	Urinary tract infection		WA	White adult
UV	Ultraviolet		WAP	Wandering atrial pacemaker
V/Q	Ventillation/perfusion ratio		WB	White boy
VA	Veterans Administration, visual acuity		WD/WN	Well developed/well nourished
VAH	Veterans Administration hospital		WF	White female
VB	Ventricular beat		WG	White girl
VC	Vena cava, vital capacity, color vision		WM	White man, male
			WNL	Within normal limits
VD	Venereal disease		WPW	Wolff-Parkinson-White)
VF	Ventricular fibrillation		wt	Weight
VG	Very good		X	times, for
VH	Ventricular hypertrophy		Y, yr.	Year
			y/o	Years old, year-old

References

Judge, R.D., Zuidema, G.D., Fitzerald, P.T., et al, *Clinical Diagnosis* 4th Edition, (Boston, MA: Little, Brown & Company, 1982).

Gazzaniga, Alan B., et al, *Emergency Care Principles & Practices for the EMT-Paramedic,* 2nd Edition, (Reston, VA, 1982).

Bledsoe, B.E., Bosker, G., Pappa, F.S., *Prehospital Emergency Pharmacology,* 2nd Edition, (Englewood Cliffs, NJ: Prentice-Hall, 1988).

Charting Symbols

The charting symbols that follow represent those that EMS personnel will most likely encounter and use. As with the section on abbreviatons, any list of charting symbols will be incomplete. Also, a symbol may be well-accepted in one region, but vitually unused in another. Including the list may tempt the user to turn his written reports into a maze of lines and dots as well as an alphabet soup of run-on abbreviations.

The listing is here as a guide. It relies on several sources for its development. If you encounter symbols not depicted here, direct your search to the listed references. Also, refer to sources such as other textbooks or a medical dictionary.

c, $\bar{c}$	[L. *cum*]. With	±	Plus or minus; either positive or negative; indefinite
Δ	Change, heat		
μg	Microgram	#	Number; following a number, pounds
mEq	Milliequivalent		
mg	Milligram	÷	Divided by
mg. %	Milligrams percent; milligrams per 100 ml.	×	Multiplied by; magnification
Po$_2$	Partial pressure of oxygen	=	Equals
Pco$_2$	Partial pressure of carbon dioxide	>	Greater than; from which is derived
$\bar{s}$	Without	<	Less than; derived from
$\bar{ss}$, ss	[L. *semis*]. One-half	≮	Not less than
		≯	Not greater than
+	Plus; excess; acid reaction; positive	≤	Equal to or less than
		≥	Equal to or greater than
–	Minus; deficiency; alkaline reaction; negative	≠	Not equal to

′	Infinity		○, ♀	Female
:	Ratio; "is to"		⇌	Denotes a reversible reaction
::	Equality between ratios; "as"		↓	Decreasing; down; lower; below
∴	Therefore		↑	Increasing; elevate; up; above
°	Degree			
%	Percent		Ⓛ	Left
□, ♂	Male		Ⓡ	Right

References

Gazzaniga, Alan B., et al, *Emergency Care Principles & Practices for the EMT-Paramedic,* 2nd Edition, (Reston, VA, 1982).

Thomas, CC (Ed.) *Taber's Cyclopedic Medical Dictionary,* 15th Edition, (Philadelphia: F.A. Davis Co., 1985)

End Notes

[1] Goldstein, AS; *EMS and the Law: A Legal Handbook for EMS Personnel*, Brady (Bowie, 1983) pages 128-129

[2] Lazar,RA;*EMS Law: A Guide for EMS Professionals*, Aspen Publishers (Rockville 1989) pages 106-107.

[3] Discussion of EMS report forms, I.C.U. staff nurses, Faulkner Hospital, Boston, MA, May 1987

[4] Ibid.

[5] Lazar,RA, *EMS Law: A Guide for EMS Professionals*,Aspen Publishers (Rockville 1989) page 108.

[6] Ibid. page 112.

[7] American Heart Association, *Textbook of Advanced Cardiac Life Support*, 2nd edition, AHA, (Dallas, 1987). page 271.

[8] Ibid. page 272.

[9] Lazar, R.A.,*EMS Law, A Guide for EMS Professionals*, (Aspen Publisher's, Inc., Rockville, 1989) pages 82-83.

[10] Berkow, Robert, Editor-in-Chief, et al, *The Merck Manual of Diagnosis and Therapy*, 14th Edition, (Merck, Sharp & Dohme Research Laboratories, Rahway, NJ; 1982). page 2231

[11] Ibid page 2231

[12] Ibid. page 2232

13 Ibid page 2231

14 Ibid. page 2233

15 Ibid. page 2233

16 Ibid. page 2233

17 Judge, R.D., Zuidema, G.D., Fitzgerald, P. T., et al,*Clinical Diagnosis* 4th Edition, (Boston, MA: Little, Brown & Company, 1982). pages 525-531.

18 Caroline, Nancy L., *Emergency Care in the Streets*, 4th Edition, (Boston, MA: Little, Brown & Company, 1991), page 257.

19 Gazzaniga, Alan B., et al, *Emergency Care Principles & Practices for the EMT-Paramedic*, 2nd Edition, (Reston, VA, 1982) page 115.

20 Budassi, S.A., Barber, J., *Mosby's Manual of Emergency Care Practices and Procedures*, 2nd Edition (St. Louis: C.V. Mosby Co., 1984). page 13.

21 Caroline, Nancy L., *Emergency Care in the Streets*, 4th Edition, (Boston: Little, Brown & Company, 1991). page 257.

22 Boyd, Kate, "The Power of Paperwork", *jems*; 5(5); (July 1980). page 22.

23 Hafen, B.Q., Karren, K.J., *Prehospital Emergency Care & Crisis Intervention*, 2nd Edition, (Englewood, CO: Morton Publishing Company, 1983). page 83.

24 Judge, R.D., Zuidema, G.D., Fitzgerald, P. T., et al, *Clinical Diagnosis*, 4th Edition, (Boston, MA: Little, Brown & Company, 1982). page 13.

25 Ibid; page 13

26 Ibid; page 14

27 Ibid; page 14

28 American Heart Association: "Standards and Guidelines for CardioPulmonary Resuscitation & Emergency Cardiac Care"; *JAMA*:

Volume 255, Number 21; June 6, 1986 page 2908

29 Judge, R.D., Zuidema, G.D., Fitzgerald, P. T., et al:*Clinical Diagnosis*: 4th Edition; Little, Brown & Company; Boston, MA; 1982 page 15

30 Shanaberger, Carol J., The Trip Report Is Important *jems*. October 1987, 12(10) pages 63-65.

31 Interviews: Anna Sinclair, M.D., Emergency Department, Quincy City Hospital, Quincy Mass. November 18, 1987, and Peter Moyer, M.D., Medical Director, Boston EMS, Boston City Hospital, Boston, Mass., November 30, 1987.

32 Interview: Anna Sinclair, M.D., Emergency Department, Quincy City Hospital, Quincy, Mass., November 11, 1987.

33 Ibid.

34 Interviews: Anna Sinclair, M.D., Emergency Department, Quincy Hospital, Quincy, Mass., November 18, 1987, and Peter Moyer, M.D., Medical Director, Boston EMS, Boston City Hospital, Boston, Mass., November 30, 1987.

35 Interview: Anna Sinclair, M.D., Emergency Department, Quincy Hospital, Quincy, Mass., November 18, 1987.

36 Shanaberger, Carol J., The Trip Report Is Important, *jems*, October 1987, 12(10), pages 63-65.

37 Ibid.

38 Cosgriff, J.H., Anderson, D.L., *The Practice of Emergency Nursing*, (Philadelphia: J.B. Lippencott Co., 1975). page 41.

39 Ellis, J.R., Hartley, C.L., *Nursing in Today's World*, 2nd Edition, (Philadelphia: J.B. Lippencott Co., 1984). page 228.

40 Caroline, Nancy L., *Emergency Medical Treatment*, (Boston, MA: Little Brown & Company, 1982). page 6.

41 Grant, H.D., Murray, R.H., Bergeron, J.D., *Emergency Care*, 4th Edition .Englewood Cliffs, NJ: Brady (Prentice-Hall), 1986. page 15.

42 American Academy of Orthopaedic Surgeons, *Emergency Care and Transportation of the Sick and Injured*, 5th Edition AAOS, (Park Ridge, IL, 1992). page 6.

43 Dernocoeur, Kate, *Streetsense*. (Bowie, MD: Brady, 1985). page 197.

44 Burgess, Ann Wolbert, *Psychiatric Nursing in the Hospital and the Community*, 4th Edition, (Englewood Cliffs, NJ: Prentice-Hall, Inc., 1985). page 674.

45 Ibid. page 674.

46 Rennert, Margot, "Sparing the Rod to Save the Child",*emergency medical services*. 15(3), 1986. page 37, 38.

47 Massachusetts General Laws (Annotated), Chapter 119, Section 51A.

48 Commonwealth of Massachusetts, Department of Social Services. Informational materials concerning child abuse.

49 Ibid.

50 Ibid.

51 Ibid

52 Ibid.

53 Ibid.

54 Burgess, Ann Wolbert, *Psychiatric Nursing in the Hospital and the Community*, 4th Edition, (Englewood Cliffs, NJ: Prentice-Hall, Inc., 1985). page 674.

55 Commonwealth of Massachusetts, Department of Social Services. Informational materials concerning child abuse.

56 Ibid.

57 Ibid.

58 Ibid.

59 Ibid.

60 Ibid.

61 Massachusetts General Laws (Annotated), Chapter 119, Section 51A.

62 Interview, Mr. James J. Connors, Case Practice Supervisor, Office for Professional Services, Commonwealth of Massachusetts, Department of Social Services, November 20, 1987.

63 Ibid.

64 Interview, Ms. Janice Powers, Commonwealth of Massachusetts, Department of Social Services, (formerly of the Boston Regional Screening Unit), November 20, 1987.

65 Stuart, CP, Elder Abuse, *Emergency Medical Services*, 20 (7) 1991 page 50

66 Ibid. page 50

67 Ibid. page 50, 68

68 Interview. Ms. Fran Joseph, Regional Supervisor, Commonwealth of Massachusetts, Executive Office of Elder Affairs, November 20, 1987.

69 Commonwealth of Massachusetts, Executive Office of Elder Affairs, Elder Abuse Brochure.

70 Moreau, D.M., *Crime Scene As A Process*, Forensic Science Training Unit, FBI Academy,(Quantico) page 20

71 Tinker, R.E.,*Crime Scene Response,*Boston Police Academy Training Bulletin 20-87.

72 Moreau, D.M., *Crime Scene As A Process*, Forensic Science Training Unit, FBI Academy,(Quantico) page 22,32

73 Ibid.,page 35

74 Goldstein, A.S.,*EMS and the Law, A Legal Handbook for EMS Personnel,*(Brady, Bowie MD) 1983; page 108

75 American Heart Association, *Textbook of Advanced Cardiac Life Support*, 2nd edition, AHA, (Dallas, 1987). page 276.

76 American Heart Association, *Textbook of Advanced Cardiac Life Support*, 2nd edition, AHA, (Dallas, 1987). pages 277-278.

77 American Heart Association, *Textbook of Advanced Cardiac Life Support*, 2nd edition, AHA, (Dallas, 1987). pages 279-283.

78 American Heart Association, *Textbook of Advanced Cardiac Life Support*, 2nd edition, AHA, (Dallas, 1987). page 276.

79 Lazar,RA, *EMS law: A Guide for EMS Professionals*, Aspen Publishers; (Rockville, 1989) pages 82–83.

80 Bonnin, M.J., Swor, R.A.; Outcomes in unsuccessful field resuscitation attemts, *Annals of Emergency Medicine*, May 1989, 18(5), pages 51–56.

81 Frank, M.; Should we terminate futile resuscitations in the field? Can we afford not to? *Annals of Emergency Medicine*, May 1989, 18(5), pages 153–155.

82 Caroline, Nancy L., *Emergency Care In The Streets*, 4th Edition, (Boston: Little Brown & Company, 1991), page 943.

83 American Heart Association, *Textbook of Advanced Cardiac Life Support*, 2nd Edition, AMA (Dallas, 1987), pages 271–272.

84 American Academy of Orthopedic Surgeons, *Emergency Care and Transportation of the Sick and Injured* 5th Edition, AAOS (Park Ridge, Illinois, 1992). page 832.

85 Cosgriff, J.H., Anderson, D.L., *The Practice of Emergency Nursing*, (Philadelphia: J.B. Lippincott Company, 1975). page 41.

86 American Academy of Orthopedic Surgeons, *Emergency Care and Transportation of the Sick*

and Injured, 5th Edition, AAOS (Park Ridge, Illinois, 1992) page 850.

87 Ibid. page 851.

88 Ibid. page 840.

89 Caroline, Nancy L. *Emergency Care In The Streets*, 4th Edition, (Boston: Little, Brown & Company, 1991). page 954.

90 American Heart Association, *Textbook of Advanced Cardiac Life Support*, 2nd Edition, AHA, (Dallas, 1987). page 279.

91 Thomas, C.L. (ed.), *Taber's Cyclopedic Medical Dictionary*, 15th Edition (Philadelphia: F.A. Davis Company, 1985), page 1001.

92 American Academy of Orthopedic Surgeons, *Emergency Care and Transportation of the Sick and Injured*, 5th Edition, AAOS (Par9k Ridge, Illinois, 1992), page 855.

93 Ibid. page 865.

Index

A

Abbreviation, 38.
    in history of present illness,
       24.
    non-standard, 24.
    table of, 185.
Abondonment
    defined, 183.
Abuse
    See Child abuse and neglect.
    See also Elder abuse.
Advanced life support
    See ALS.
Allergies, 25.
    vs. side effects, 25.
ALS, 11, 27, 36, 76, 84 – 85.

B

Belligerent patient, 60.
Billing information, 12.
BLS, 84 – 85, 160 – 161, 163, 169 –
171, 173 – 174.
Breach of duty
    defined, 183.

C

Cases
    used in classroom exercises,
       159 – 160.
Cause of death, 76.

Changes during transport,
    27 – 28.
Charting symbols
    table of, 195.
Chief complaint, 21 – 22, 38.
Child abuse and neglect, 61 – 62.
    characteristics of abusive
       persons, 62.
    Child Abuse Prevention and
Treatment Act, 61.
    Child At Risk Hotline, 65.
    Child-At-Risk Hotline, 65.
    mandated reporters, 61, 66.
    Massachusetts general laws,
       61.
    mechanism of injury, 63.
    neglect, 64.
    physical indicators, 62 – 63.
    stage of development factor,
       63.
    statistics, 65.
Classroom exercises, 159 – 175.
    cases used in, 159 – 160.
CMR records, 179.
Common deficiencies in report
writing, 177 – 178.
Consent, 55.
    actual consent, 183.
    defined, 183.
    implied, 183.
    informed, 183.
    informed consent, 55.

withdrawal of, 56.
Crime scene, 72.
    evidence reported by EMS
        personnel, 72.
    management of, 69 – 70.
    regarding sudden death, 75.
    summons issued to any
        person present, 70.

D

Disagreement
    with medical control
        technician, 42.
DNR
    See Do not resuscitate orders.
Do not resuscitate order
    imminence of death, 73.
    patient competency, 73.
Do not resuscitate orders, 72 –
74.
Drug administration
    See Medicine, administration
        of.
Duty to act
    defined, 184.
Duty to perform
    defined, 184.

E

ECG
    See Electrocardiogram.
EKG
    See Electrocardiogram.
Elder abuse, 67 – 68.
    Elder Abuse Hotline, 68.
    indications of, 68.
    mandated reporters, 68.
    Massachusetts law, 68.
Electrocardiogram, 27, 42, 161,
    168.

Emergency department staff, 51,
    54.
Emergency room
    presenting your case in,
        51.
EMT
    as an extension of the
        physician, 13, 50.

F

Family history, 25.
Findings
    from physical examination, 26.

G

Goals, 9.

H

History of present illness, 22, 38.
    inclusions/exclusions, 23.
    use of abbreviation, 24.
Hospital resources
    run report as, 41.

I

I.V., 27, 36, 42, 56, 161, 163,
    165 – 166, 169 – 171.
Implied consent, 183.
Informed consent, 55.
    defined, 55, 183.
Informed refusal, 57.
Intubation, 27.
Investigating complaints
    Mass. Department of Public
Health, 181.
Investigation
    of complaints, 181.

L

Law
105 CMR 170.240 Records, 179.
accuracy of abbreviation, 24.
concerning child abuse and neglect, 61.
contractual agreement, 13.
documenting suddent death, 75.
implied contract, 13.
legal documents, 12.
liability and malpractice, 13.
malpractice claim substantiation, 13.
malpractice defined, 184.
Massachusetts regarding elder abuse, 68.
medical legal, 12.
Negligence defined, 184.
Reporting procedure, abuse/neglect in Mass., 65.
Legal documents, 12.
Liability and malpractice, 13 – 14.
contractual agreement, 13.
implied contract, 13.
malpractice claim substantiation, 13.

M

Malpractice
defined, 184.
See Liability and malpractice.
Mandated reports
of elder abuse, 68.
Massachusetts Department of Public Health
Office of Emergency Medical Services, 181.
Mechanism of injury, 41.

in child abuse, 63.
Medical control
speaking with, 48.
Medical control physician, 48, 50.
Medical record, 12.
Medical-legal, 12.
Medication, 41.
administration of, 42.
recording effects of, 41.
Modified problem/source medical record, 16.

N

Neglect
See Child abuse and neglect.
Negligence
defined, 184.
Non-transport situation, 59.
Notification, 46.

P

Past medical history, 25.
family history, 25.
risk factors, 25.
social history, 25.
Patient
belligerent, 60.
Patient refusals, 57.
Physical examination, 26, 47.
Physical findings, 51.
PMH
See Past Medical History.
Problem oriented reporting format, 15.
Problem/Source reporting format, 16.
Proper documentation, 41.

Q

Quality of service, 14.

R

Radio communication, 54.
    advising patient of, 56.
    ambulance-to-hospital,
        45 – 46.
Refusal
    documenting, 58 – 59.
    informed, 57.
Report form, 11.
Report writing
    common deficiencies,
        177 – 178.
    point to remember, 38.
    points to remember, 39.
Reporting formats, 15.
    problem oriented medical
record, 15.
    problem/source, 16.
    S.O.A.P., 16.
    SEMS (Simplified EMS)
        format, 19.
    SEMS format, 20.
    source oriented, 16.
    traditional write-up, 17.
Research, 12.
Rights
    right to refuse medical
        treatment, 57.
Risk factors, 25.
Run reports, 83.
    as a hospital resource, 41.
    as a valuable resource, 42.

S

S.O.A.P. reporting format, 16.
    assessment, 16.
    objective findings, 16.
    plan, 16.

subjective findings, 16.
SEMS format, 19 – 20, 49,
    51 – 52.
    changes during transport,
        27 – 28.
    chief complaint, 21 – 22.
    history of present illness, 22.
    in ambulance-to-hospital
        radio communication, 47.
    past medical history (PMH),
        25.
    physical examination, 26.
    treatment given, 26 – 27.
    use of, 20.
Simplified EMS format
    See SEMS format.
Social history, 25.
Source oriented reporting
    format, 16.
Special reporting situations, 55.
    consent, 55.
Standard of care
    defined, 184.
Statistics, 12.
Sudden death
    cause of death, 76.
    crime scene management, 75.
    documentation used in
        litigation, 77.
    effort to resusciate terminated
        pre-transport, 75.
    medical-legal documentation,
        76.
    no effort to resuscitate, 75.
Suddent death, 74.
    documenting, 74.
Symbols
    table of charting symbols, 195.

T

Traditional write-up reporting
    format, 17.

Treatment, 46, 48.
Treatment given, 26 – 27.
    administering medications, 27.
Triage, 46 – 47, 51.
    process, 52.
Triage systems, 45.

V

Vital signs
    changes in, 26.
    recording, 26.

W

Withdrawal of consent, 56.
Witnesses, 59.
Written reports
    purpose, form, & content, 11.

Additional copies of this text can be obtained by calling customer service toll free at:

1-877 288 4737

or visit our web site at:

www.iUniverse.com

iUniverse.com
toExcel Press/Publishing Services
620 North 48th Street, Suite 201
Lincoln, Nebraska 68504-3467